VOLUME 1: AWAKEN

Food and Intuition 101

JULIA FERRÉ

May the Light Within You Shine....

Other Books by Julia Ferré
Basic Macrobiotic Cooking
Food and Intuition 101 Volume 2: Developing Intuition
French Meadows Cookbook

Edited by Kathy Keller
Cover and text design by Carl Ferré

First Edition   2012 May 31
Current Edition, minor edits   2013 Mar 23

Published with the help of East West Center for Macrobiotics
    www.EastWestMacrobiotics.com

ISBN 978-0-918860-71-2

Preface

The goal of this book is to empower you to thrive—to have physical vitality, emotional stability, and spiritual involvement. Then, you can make informed choices, have conviction about those choices, and be tolerant of the choices of others.

The book allows you to learn in your own home, do your own cooking, and move at your own pace. You are free to eat whatever diet you choose, make whatever decisions feel right for you, and succeed in whatever situations you find yourself.

Although this book is about intuition, it didn't start out that way. Since 1980, I have cooked food according to macrobiotic ideas, written one cookbook, compiled another, and helped run a yearly summer gathering where people camp outdoors and eat whole, plant-based foods. Initially, I wanted to write about food based on these experiences.

Before I began to write, I meditated to clear my mind. The ideas that emerged were different from what I anticipated. The first ten lessons weren't about cooking at all! They were about how we relate to food, how we choose to be healthy, how we choose to take care of ourselves, and how we choose food based on thinking. Over the next three months, I meditated every day. Gradually, the outline for this book became clear.

Using the tools in this book, you can change your life—based on your uniqueness and individual needs. Comprehensive guidelines help you determine healthy dietary choices, cultivate your unconscious, and facilitate your intuition. Unlike navigating complex approaches focused on health, weight loss, animal rights, and so on, when you rely on your intuition, you make choices based on internal guidance rather than the latest trend.

There is no doubt in my mind that we are spiritual beings who live in physical bodies. Intuition is being in touch with this state. This book will help you understand that intuition is a valuable part of your life and strengthen your connection with it.

I offer you the best of luck and well wishes as you incorporate these lessons into your life.

Julia Ferré
April 2012

Contents

Acknowledgments

Thank you to the following individuals who helped in the publication of this book:

Carl Ferré, my husband, who not only listened patiently to various ideas, lessons, and exercises since the inception of the book but also worked tirelessly in seeing the book through to completion; Kathy Keller, my editor, who clarified what needed to be clarified, removed what needed to be removed, and added what needed to be added; and close friends, Sandy Rothman, Saci McDonald, and Bob Ligon, who read parts of the manuscript and provided valuable feedback and support.

I also value friends who offered encouragement over the years: Barbara and Michael Brown, Claudia Delman, Tim Galanek, Barb Jurecki, Rebekah Karlen, Dawn Pallavi Ludwig, Ann Polivka, Charlotte Rainwater, surrogate mother Mary, and all the women in my women's group.

I express love to my kids, Gus, Nels, Franz, and John, for their love and support in return, and to my teacher and mentor, Athena, who continues to be my muse and provide inspiration and advice.

Introduction

Everyone is born with intuition. It begins with your first breath and develops throughout your life. An automatic inner knowing and feeling, intuition indicates the right thing to do. It is innate, personal, practical, and immediate. You can cultivate your intuition to help you thrive and live the life you want.

Intuition is like a guiding compass for finding satisfaction and avoiding pain. It aids us across a broad spectrum—from caring for basic needs and deriving pleasure in life to searching for meaningful relationships and fulfilling careers.

A lot of what we consider intuition is actually learned behavior. For example, the other day I was filling a glass of water from the tap. Because the room was dim, I couldn't see when the glass was full. But, I could hear the sound of the glass filling and knew when to turn off the water before the glass overflowed. At first, I considered this to be intuition. On second thought, I realized it was learned behavior. At some age, I had learned the differing sounds of water as a glass becomes full. Now, I rely on this knowledge to know when to turn off the tap. Another example is when we say we intuitively like or dislike something or someone. Often, our feelings are based on our previous interactions and experiences with the thing or person.

Intuition is part of our innate intelligence that is reinforced through trial and error and refined by associations we form. Physical manifestations of intuition include instincts, reflexes, and the needs for sleep, nourishment, and love. For example, humans (like other mammals) are born with certain requirements: to drink, to eat, to sleep, to be close to others. We learn to find water, food, shelter, companionship. Over time, we learn to store water, prepare food, make more secure abodes, and cultivate relationships. Using our senses to understand the world and our intuition to guide us, we further develop our abilities to survive and thrive.

Not everyone is aware of his or her intuition. This book can help you become more aware of your intuition, where it already flourishes within you, and how to awaken or enhance other intuitive abilities.

Intuition and Food Support Each Other

There are a number of reasons why food is useful in understanding and developing intuition:

1. Food is universal; we have to eat every day. Unlike meditation, another practical method to understand and foster intuition, food is not optional. Regular eating is a reliable resource for learning, especially given the frequent opportunities to practice.

2. Food is unique and personal. Incorporating it in the study of intuition makes the subject individually interesting.

3. Food is the foundation for living. We eat in order to survive, which allows us to thrive by doing all the other things we want. Attitudes and habits formed in our basic relationship to food affect our perceptions and actions in other areas of our lives.

4. Food affects our health and emotions. In turn, physical health affects how our mind operates, while emotions color our thinking.

5. Food has a direct relationship to health, appearance, and sense of worth. Currently, many people are challenged with out-of-control addictions or non-supportive attitudes about food and self-identity. Learning about healthy food, healthy attitudes, and how intuition shapes healthy choices is the foundation for relating to food in a meaningful way.

6. Intuition, like food, is something everyone has; both may be utilized consciously. Like food, intuition can be developed to an art.

7. Intuition and food interact: intuition helps one choose healthy food; the strong body, mind, and spirit derived from eating healthy food makes the intuitive ability stronger.

Most people want to eat in a healthy way, but they are exposed to countless diets and theories about food...what to eat and what to avoid. Navigating this information is easier when we use our intuition because it helps us choose the foods that satisfy us and formulate a diet that supports us.

How to Use This Book

This is Volume 1 of *Food and Intuition 101*. It introduces techniques to help you 1) become aware of the intuition already present within you and 2) apply this intuitive ability to selecting and preparing food with confidence. The long-term goal is to instill healthy habits within you based on your own needs and preferences.

This book contains 42 lessons grouped in units of six lessons each, with a theme for each unit. These sequential lessons are intended to be followed in order from 1 to 42. Within each group of lessons, your relationship to food is explored—from selection and preparation to consumption. Culinary techniques are discussed, as well as how to choose quality foods and equipment. Some recipes and menus are also included.

It is intended that you do one lesson per day, completing one unit each week. However, take whatever time you need or desire. If you need a break, it is best to take it between units to maintain continuity within each unit. I suggest you not attempt more than one lesson a day and that you not skip lessons or jump ahead because the lessons build on each other to provide a foundation of understanding. Do your best—willingness is preferred; perfection is not required.

In Volume 2 of *Food and Intuition 101*, you will develop your intuition further. The second volume continues by introducing and explaining, in depth, seven areas of intuition with numerous exercises that apply intuition to food and beyond. The two volumes comprise a course of 101 individual lessons.

Use this course as a tool to help raise your own intuitive awareness and to become healthier. There is no expectation for you to become a vegetarian, macrobiotic, vegan, or any other kind of "diet-identified" person, now, or for the rest of your life. However, it is my hope that this manual will help you integrate positive changes that fit your needs for the rest of your life. This, to me, is putting your intuition to work.

Reclaiming Intuition

Health and intuition are related. Often, pain, disease, and stress are promptings to seek relief. These promptings signal that intuition is at work. A healthy body is free from pain that impedes clear thoughts. The healthier a person is, the easier it is to cultivate intuition.

While everyone has inner signals, not everyone knows how to interpret them. In addition, there are some situations that hamper intuitive ability, such as the following:

1. Addictions that interfere with and hide an accurate internal awareness.

2. Extreme childhood traumas that result in not trusting one's internal voice.

3. Extreme betrayal that results in not trusting others or advice in general.

4. Assumptions and second guessing such as feeling that you should have avoided a natural disaster or should have known better.

5. Doubt about yourself.

6. Fear, an emotion that always creates confusion and chaos.

7. Embarrassment due to prior situations.

Awakening Intuition

This book presents information about how intuition is naturally present within each person and provides exercises to help the reader become fully in touch with intuition. Here are suggestions to reclaim intuition and to help awaken it and its fullest potential:

1. Overcome addiction. Addiction can be serious, and you should seek counsel from a reputable doctor or therapist if needed. While this book offers simple advice for simple addictions, it is not a substitute for qualified care for serious addictions.

2. Educate yourself. Information elevates the mind.

3. Perform exercises to apply the information. You need both theoretical understanding and practical work.

4. Establish healthy habits. It is vital to install rhythm and orderliness in taking care of basic needs, including food, physical exercise, and rest.

5. Practice safety and common sense as much as you can.

6. Be positive. Create as much positive force in your life as possible.

7. See the bigger picture. Cultivate trust in the positive side of life.

Intuition, I feel, is a natural inborn ability that can help you see how you do things right. I am sure of this. You, like most everyone on the planet, seek to do things correctly, and I believe intuition is the process behind it. This course centers on that idea—that you do things right.

May your intuition help you thrive and be empowered in your physical vitality, emotional stability, mental integrity, and spiritual awareness.

Start Where You Are

Start where you are, my friends. Now is the place to be. You already do things that are healthy; you already take care of yourself; you already do things that are intuitive. Recognize these habits and attitudes and build on them to help your intuition flourish.

Stop, reflect, and appreciate where you are at this point in your life… a culmination of all your past experiences, of all your future hopes. Right now, the center of this spectrum, is the best place to evaluate what you know, how you do things, and where you are.

Keyword: Healthy

The main objective of this unit is to become aware of what you consider "healthy" food and recognize how much you rely on your intuition to make that determination. You rely on your intuition all the time for basic needs: water, food, shelter, and survival. Use your intuition when you select what to keep on your shelves and what to eat. Recognize that your intuition is the foundation of existence and is an invaluable guide in your journey to optimal health.

Food: Eat Healthy Foods

Do your best to consume "healthy" foods according to your own definition. Prepare, cook, and eat these foods, using what you have on hand, and relying on your own integrity to feed yourself well.

Exercise: Evaluate Food on Hand

Evaluate all the food you presently have in your house. Do this exercise as you progress through these six lessons. Look at everything in your cupboards, refrigerator, pantry, basement, and all other food storage places. Be as thorough as you can by applying the following steps as you go through your food supplies:

1. Relax with this exercise and have fun. There are no food police lurking in the corners so don't make this an exhausting chore. In fact, reorganizing cupboards can be invigorating.

2. Discard the worst offenders, especially moldy food, packaged goods past the expiration dates, and foods you consider "really bad." If you have dried goods such as flour or dried leafy herbs that are older than a year, compost or toss them. Flour becomes rancid, herbs lose their flavor, and packaged goods have optimal usage dates. Donate to a food bank any items that are still good but that you don't want to eat.

3. Classify the remaining foods as healthy or not-so-healthy. Some foods may be obvious—others more complicated. For this step, pay attention to the criteria you use to sort or classify items. Remember: whatever classification criteria you use is valid. The point of this exercise is to recognize that you already have ideas about which foods are good for you and which foods are not.

   When I last did this exercise, I had to reconsider products with multiple ingredients (some healthy, others not); foods marketed as "good;" specialty foods required for holidays or guests; and foods for other members in the household.

4. Sort and group items by whatever criteria make sense to you. Perhaps you place all bottled items or snack items together. Maybe individual members of the house have their

own shelf space. Perhaps put items that you want to use first in a certain area so you can replace them with healthier options after finished.

5. Use your intuition to choose foods that nourish. Whether a food is packaged, bulk, fresh, or canned is not as important as whether or not you consider it beneficial to your health and worth consuming.

Resources: Appendix 1
◊ *Intuition about Shopping*

Getting Started: Lessons 1 to 6
Start by examining your basic relationship to food. Learn to appreciate the gift of food, to spend quality time with food. In the process, you become increasingly aware of what *healthy* means to you when applied to food. Pace yourself well in practicing the following six lessons. Apply only one lesson each day and do your best to feed yourself well. This will help you put the lessons into practice and strengthen your basic relationship to food and intuition.

Lesson 1

The Miracle of Life

Life is a miracle; you are a miracle!

How amazing that humans can walk, talk, and move—thanks to a body that can breathe, think, and interact! When we contemplate the complexity of our bodies, we understand that life is nothing short of a miracle! Without much effort, we breathe, wake, move, and consume. Nonetheless, human life exists on the planet in only very specific conditions: to live, we need light, oxygen, water, and food.

Some species, such as dinosaurs, became extinct when their food supply dwindled. The same thing could happen to panda bears if their sole source of nourishment (bamboo) disappeared. Fortunately, we are not limited to one specific food. Instead, as a highly adaptive species, humans are able to consume a far great diversity of foods than most other species. We can survive on meat, vegetables, fish, or simply junk food. Although far from optimal, a human could subsist on junk food alone.

In most modern societies, food is abundant and, although an essential element for life, it is generally taken for granted. Yet, anyone who has lived in poverty, has had to ration food during war or emergencies, or has simply run out of food while camping does not take food for granted.

All food intended for human consumption, whether animal or vegetal, is meant to nourish. There is considerable debate about the merits of animal versus vegetal foods and the quality of life each generates. And some individuals even develop life-threatening allergies to particular foods. Nonetheless, all food has the capacity to nourish—organically grown or not, animal or vegetal, carbohydrate or fat or protein.

Exercise 1: The Gift of Food

Each time you eat today, focus on food as nourishment.

At any particular meal, thoroughly chew three mouthfuls of any one food you consider *healthy*—it can be vegetable, grain, protein, or fruit. The choice of the food does not matter as much as whether or not you consider it to be a "healthy" food.

For the first bite, pay special attention to the taste of the food and count the number of times you chew that mouthful. For the second bite, continue to concentrate on the taste of the food and increase the number of times you chew that mouthful. If you chewed the first bite 20 times, chew the second bite 30 times. For the third bite, increase the number of chews by ten again. Each time, savor the food and reflect on how it provides nourishment to your body. For the rest of the meal, you don't need to count the number of times you chew each mouthful, although you can if you wish.

Summary

Food is nourishment for the body. When you slow down and focus on each bite of food while eating, your intuition is heightened and you realize how important food is to your life.

Lesson 2

Hunger

Hunger keeps you alive. Understand your hunger to tune into your intuition.

Hunger is a basic and powerful instinct; it is present in a newborn infant who knows immediately how to suckle without being taught. I witnessed this firsthand when I put my babies at my breast within minutes of birth. Each one latched on and began sucking, even though no milk was yet present.

During the first months of life, an infant must suckle to live. If the baby lacks the ability or strength to suckle, it will die—unless there is an intervention. Also innately, a baby cries when hungry to signal it needs to be fed.

Initially, a newborn baby's hunger has no pattern, day or night. Over time, hunger becomes strongest in the morning, around noon, and in the evening. A rhythm develops and eventually becomes breakfast, lunch, and dinner. As adults, we maintain these routines, which if interrupted, provoke a response. Skip a meal, and the stomach growls.

Hunger is your inborn desire for food; it is a drive for nourishment and different from appetite. Think of how you feel when you are physically exhausted and need to eat; almost any food is appealing. Appetite, on the other hand, is a desire for specific food items. Think of seeing an image of delicious food that makes your mouth water. This is appetite, the fun response to food.

Your hunger keeps you alive and should not be taken for granted. You can use your drive to eat as a foundation for health. Indeed, working with your hunger is one of the building blocks of this book.

Exercise 2: Receiving Food

In this exercise, we build on the first lesson: how food sustains life. Today, we focus on how hunger, the desire for food, supports the gift of life.

At any two meals or snack times, consciously chew three bites of any food you consider healthy. As before, count the number of chews for each bite, extending the number for the second and third bites. This time, think about your relationship with food and determine whether this particular food is satisfying your *hunger* or your *appetite*.

Summary

At its most basic, hunger is an innate drive to find food to fill the belly. It differs from appetite, which can be highly selective. At the same time, hunger and appetite are not exclusive to food. They can reflect a drive for greater satisfaction. For example, we hunger for adventure, have an appetite for a fulfilling career, or yearn for meaningful relationships. Let your hunger guide you toward nourishment of both your body and your spirit. Paying attention to what you hunger for helps you tune into your intuition.

Lesson 3

Breathing

Breathing establishes life. Breathe when you eat, and breathe life into your intuitive relationship with food.

At birth, a child takes its first breath and lives—able for the first time to survive without its mother. Breathing is a simple process of moving air in and out of the lungs. Without conscious effort, it delivers oxygen to where it is needed in the body and removes carbon dioxide. Breathing soon becomes automatic, unless there is an incident or trauma, and eventually, it too is taken for granted.

You can benefit from heightened awareness of your breathing, as emphasized by yoga and other disciplines that stress the importance of inhaling deeply to increase lung capacity and exhaling completely to empty the lungs. Beyond these basics, you can learn other techniques that cultivate relaxation and rejuvenation through advanced breathing exercises that aim to integrate body, mind, and spirit.

There is a parallel between breathing and chewing. Just as breathing is the means to access the oxygen in air, chewing is the means to access the nutrition in food. When you chew, you grind food into increasingly smaller pieces that, when mixed with saliva, make food nutrients available to be assimilated by your body. Similarly, when you breathe, you assimilate elements found in air (nitrogen, oxygen, etc.) that nourish your body by metabolism of energy-rich molecules such as glucose. Breathing, like chewing, is automatic and often taken for granted. Yet, like chewing, breathing can be used consciously to enhance health and raise awareness.

Exercise 3: Observation of Eating

Evaluate your eating by consciously breathing and chewing simultaneously.

For this exercise, eat at least three different healthy foods at one meal. At the beginning of the meal, chew one mouthful of the first dish as long as possible and, if helpful, count your number of chews. Breathe regularly while chewing and evaluate the dish in whatever ways become apparent. Consider the food in a simple and light-hearted way. First, you may think of the taste and texture, or who made the dish, and then where the food was grown, or how it agrees with you.

Evaluate the next dish in a similar way and observe any differences or similarities to the first dish. Perhaps one dish appeals to you more than the other. Be aware of your responses, and be comfortable with whatever information comes to you. This exercise is one of becoming aware, not of critiquing food. After the exercise, proceed with the rest of the meal in your usual fashion.

Summary

Your response to food is individual and unique. When you take time to breathe and reflect while eating, you are using your intuition.

Lesson 4

Respect

You have a complex and long-lasting relationship with food—a relationship you cannot live without. When you respect this relationship, you raise your consciousness and increase your intuition about food, as well as about other areas in your life.

Throughout history, people have demonstrated respect for food. Many cultures serve traditional dishes for holidays or perform ceremonial food rituals. Some people plant and harvest foods with special prayers or perform dances to honor the rhythms of nature. Nowadays, respect for food is often demonstrated by saying grace before a meal, pausing to appreciate the bounty of food. But, true respect for food is more than a simple "thank you."

Consider the respect we feel toward people such as the Dalai Lama and Mother Teresa, students who earn PhDs or black belts in karate, or people who achieve outstanding goals. We honor people who live to be 100, couples who celebrate many years of marriage, and individuals who master an art or craft. A common theme in these examples is that these accomplishments require time. Usually, the degree of our respect is in proportion to the amount of time the individual spent on the effort.

Now, consider the amount of time you devote to eating. If you counted the hours—not to mention time spent gardening, shopping, and cooking—you would be surprised. Consider whether you've spent as much time on any other activity over the course of your lifetime, day in, day out, working or on vacation, alone or with others, without fail. Sleeping, perhaps; breathing, of course…but these are activities we perform without thought. Given the tremendous amount of time you've spent developing your long-lasting relationship with food, it certainly deserves your respect!

To demonstrate your respect for food, work to acknowledge your relationship, learn about food and your health, and know your specific needs and preferences. Spend time with food and develop knowledge that forms the basis of your intuition, which will deepen over time.

Exercise 4: Time with Food

At the beginning of each meal, pause to say a grace, either a simple mental "thank you for this food" or a specific prayer of blessing or gratitude. While eating each meal, reflect on how wonderful it is to take time to eat. Make this a comfortable meal: Take only one mouthful of each dish at a time; chew each bite well; eat consciously yet in a relaxed manner; experience all that food does for you. Ideally, eat each meal this way; spend time with your food as a form of respect.

Summary

Food can help you learn about intuition because it is practical. As you learn about food, yourself, and the role of intuition in your life, practical daily experiences reinforce the lessons. Practice is a form of respect; it means doing the work, applying the lessons, living the learning, thereby reinforcing intuition.

Lesson 5

Chewing

Chewing is Zen-like. Practice becoming one with your food.

Chewing is a discipline that helps you learn about food, use food well, and spend quality time with food. It can seem like a mundane activity, and most people do chew without thinking about it. Yet, chewing thoughtfully has tremendous benefits; the greatest one is becoming truly present. In this state, you can begin to change and allow your body, emotions, mind, and spirit to thrive. Here are some ideas for you to "chew."

Physically, chewing:

1. *Breaks food down.* Breaking food into smaller pieces of food creates a larger surface area, thus facilitating absorption of nutrients by the small intestine.

2. *Eases digestion.* Smaller particles of food are easier for the "toothless" stomach to process and then pass on to the intestines.

3. *Activates saliva.* Saliva, which contains an enzyme (ptyalin) that begins the digestion of carbohydrates, coats and moistens particles of food. Complex carbohydrates are then broken into less-complex chains. A side benefit: the longer you chew carbohydrate-rich food, the more delicious it tastes.

4. *Provides alkalinity.* Saliva is alkaline, which buffers the acidity that carbohydrates produce in the body. Lengthy chewing is especially effective in creating an alkaline state.

5. *Increases food quantity.* By hydration, saliva increases the bulk of food so that we are satiated more quickly. As a result, we eat less food.

6. *Limits consumption of non-ideal foods.* If you thoroughly chew a bite of food that is less than ideal, you are less likely to eat a second bite.

7. *Lessens extreme reactions to food.* Chewing a cold item well will warm it and prevent a shock to the stomach. Similarly, thoroughly chewing foods that tend to produce intestinal bloating or gas reduces this effect. Chewing well also reduces minor allergic reactions. I am sensitive to dairy products and tomatoes; if I chew such foods well, my reactions are lessened.

8. *Exercises muscles and stimulates glands and nerves.* In addition to exercising the muscles of the jaw and face, chewing also massages glands under the neck and behind the ears while it also stimulates nerves that extend to the brain. The lymph glands then produce more beneficial secretions.

9. *Builds a foundation for health.* Over time, chewing, along with a healthy diet, positively impacts our blood, nerves, muscles, internal organs, and brain function increasing our

stamina, emotional stability, sexual vitality, and spiritual awareness in the process. Overall, chewing builds a foundation for optimal health.

Emotionally, chewing:

1. *Provides calm during meals.* Chewing slowly is a soothing exercise that helps you focus on your food.

2. *Provides calm in your long-term condition.* Thoroughly chewing healthy food on a regular basis provides more stable blood sugar, calmer moods, and increased health.

3. *Prevents overeating.* If you tend to overeat in times of stress, chewing your food well will calm you down and help you focus on what is happening. This will help you control how much you eat.

Mentally, chewing:

1. *Enhances mental function.* Movement of your jaw muscles is said to stimulate brain activity, thereby increasing your focus and making your thinking more acute.

2. *Balances mental needs.* Slow chewing calms the mind; quick chewing stimulates it. For example, when I am stressed, slow chewing provides a methodical approach to eating that is calming. When I am tired or unfocused, quick chewing provides an energetic approach that is stimulating.

3. *Enhances mental acuity.* Chewing brings you to the present moment so your powers of evaluation become more accurate, particularly in regard to non-ideal foods and difficult situations. Chewing also helps reduce reactive behavior. Wonder why you reach for that second helping of cake? Chew the first helping well and figure out why.

Spiritually, chewing:

1. *Brings awareness during meals.* It is possible to chew only

one mouthful at a time. Counting the number of times you chew each mouthful helps you focus on the present. This can be a meditative exercise.

2. *Brings awareness to your long-term condition.* The strong body, stable emotions, and focused mind that result from chewing are tools that aid your personal and spiritual growth. These tools are unending in application.

3. *Brings awareness of food and what it offers.* Slow chewing makes you more aware; as awareness increases so does gratitude.

Exercise 5: Chewing

Continue the art of taking time to eat. Sit for each of your meals today (or at least one), eat dishes that you consider healthy, and thoroughly chew at least one mouthful from each dish. Pause to enjoy the food and fully appreciate the meal.

Apply the following four ideas while you eat to enhance your physical body, emotions, mental function, and spiritual needs:

1. Chew…and digest your meal.
2. Chew…and calm your emotions.
3. Chew…and contemplate the food and your condition.
4. Chew…and appreciate all food offers you.

Summary

Chewing is an art form—always available and always appropriate. Whenever you eat, you will have the chance to chew well. Never will there be a lack of opportunity to practice. If you are rushed to eat and can't take the time to chew, be easy on yourself. Then take advantage of the opportunity at the next meal.

Learn about food—what it does and can do—and then when you eat, chew well, contemplate, and assimilate. Let food teach you, heal you, and strengthen your intuition.

Lesson 6

REVIEW: **Start Where You Are**

Stand back and appreciate who you are!
You are wonderful, full of life, and worthy
of love, appreciation, and respect.

Life is a journey from birth to death, and each day is another step along the way. Each day provides opportunities to experience and grow. Because we eat every day, we have many opportunities to learn by using eating to advance our knowledge. Each meal is an opportunity to practice; each mouthful can be a chance to learn. Don't be concerned if you aren't always able to chew consciously, take time to sit and eat, or eat healthy food; another opportunity will come—you will eat again.

This is a day to review and assess the five lessons of Unit 1 whose theme is "Start where you are." These lessons are about your basic relationship to food. Here are summaries:

Lesson 1: Life. The food you eat is one of the substances that sustains your life.

Lesson 2: Hunger. Having a desire for food is a force that keeps you alive. Because everyone gets hungry, this lesson also gives a glimpse of how intuition manifests in everyone's life.

Lesson 3: Breathing. Breathing is necessary for living. Similarly chewing is important to extract nutrients from food. Breathe consciously while eating.

Lesson 4: Respect. Respect the time to eat and respect the fact that food nourishes you and has for your whole life.

Lesson 5: Chewing. There are many benefits to be derived from thorough and thoughtful chewing—physically, emotionally, mentally, and spiritually

Use your exercise time today (and every day) to make a commitment to start where you are—each mouthful and each meal—with focus and belief that you are helping yourself. *Start where you are.* There are no other conditions or prerequisites.

Exercise 6: Mindfulness at Each Meal

Be mindful each time you eat. For meals that are rushed, such as in public or at work, simply be aware of the fact that you are eating and relish at least one bite.

For meals that are more leisurely, sit for the entire meal and take time to be present with your food. Chew at least one mouthful of each dish consciously, counting the number of chews, if needed, to help you focus. You can chew each mouthful to a count of 100 for more condensed dishes like grains, beans, and breads, if you like.

Summary

The ideas presented in these first lessons and exercises help you recognize your basic relationship to food. The simple acts of sitting, chewing, reflecting, and enjoying are foundational to this recognition. Through the rest of this book, we will build on this foundation to further your awareness and enhance your intuition, which is the cornerstone of your existence.

Unit 2

IMPETUS TO CHANGE

*Don't be afraid of change; change is just another word
for growth. Your intuition can help you make decisions
so that the change is for the best.*

In this unit, you consider how to embrace change by evaluating various ways to reinforce your basic trust in life. You learn about rhythm, habits, and how you make up your mind, and you review any experience or catalyst that urged you to change. This unit's lessons encourage you to consider the positive value of change and how to determine valid criteria for making beneficial changes.

Keyword: Trust

The main objective of this unit is to learn to trust yourself: to know that you are doing the right things to help yourself; that you have intuition; that you can use your intuition for positive guidance in making desirable changes. You'll realize that what you know now may be used as a springboard for change.

Food: Selection, Preparation, and Consumption

Three steps—selection, preparation, and consumption—are necessary components of your relationship with food. You select appropriate sources of food, prepare the food well, and then thoughtfully eat the food. Intuition plays a role in all three activities. For meals during this unit, consume healthy foods, using your definition of "healthy," and incorporate the ideas that follow. Consult *Appendix 2* for extra resources.

Exercise: Increase Your Involvement

Increase your involvement in food selection and preparation. Follow these guidelines to select and prepare food:

1. *Select food.* Search for quality food such as fresh, organic vegetables and organic whole grains. Look for stores and suppliers such as natural food stores, cooperatives, health food stores, mail-order stores, farmers' markets, and organic sections in large supermarkets. This is a wonderful way to exercise intuition, by locating businesses that sell healthy food.

2. *Prepare food.* Cooking is the best, easiest, and quickest way to develop an intuitive sense about food. By cooking, you learn about meal planning, organization, timing, flavors, and nutrition. You also learn about energy and how food creates vitality. You will learn what agrees with you or what does not. You will even learn from your mistakes. Cook for yourself at least one day during this unit. If by chance you are ill and not able to stand at the stove, at least go into the kitchen while food is being prepared and witness the activity.

3. *Consume food.* Continue to eat your meals consciously. As an aid, note on a calendar the meals when you sat and consciously chewed at least one mouthful. This practice will help you track your progress.

Resources: Appendix 2

◊ *Basic Menus*
◊ *Intuition about Cooking*
◊ *Intuition about Grains*
◊ *Intuition about Beans*
◊ *Intuition about Nuts and Seeds*
◊ *Intuition about Vegetables and Fruits*

Getting Started: Lessons 7 to 12

Change happens; it is an inevitable part of life. You know it occurs, and you trust that you will get through it. This unit emphasizes
having trust and confidence that you can respond to change, and that
the way you respond is important.

These six lessons set the foundation and pace for all the other
lessons in the book. Perfection is not required—only a willingness to
do your best. The secret is that you must do your own work. No one
can choose your habits, make you learn things, or force a change of
thinking. You must do these things yourself, with a focus on yourself. When you do, you exercise intuition and ultimately gain lasting
benefits.

A Note about Change: It takes about six weeks of daily effort
to effect a desired change, to reverse bad habits and/or create new
ones. Your mind and body need time to adjust, rewire, and establish
your new habit. Two things are required for your change to become
permanent: 1) Practice long enough for the new activity to become
habitual; 2) Undertake the change for positive reasons. Only when
the change is worthwhile will you be motivated to maintain it.

Lesson 7

Rhythm

*Intuition has its roots in the rhythms of life. When
you acknowledge and align your habits with these
rhythms, intuition becomes more active.*

Intuition begins in utero with the baby's exposure to its first sounds:
the mother's heartbeat that sets a rhythm of life—a pulse of constancy,
day and night. After birth, the mother's heartbeat continues to soothe

the baby, who is comforted simply by being close to the mother and her heartbeat.

At birth, a newborn is helpless and can do only one thing: suckle, an instinct to obtain nourishment. By the third month of life, an infant usually has settled into rhythms of eating and sleeping, resting and wakefulness that will satisfy his or her growing needs and, hopefully, mirror the habits of the caretakers. Gradually, as the baby grows, these rhythms provide stability and continuity that will persist through school years and into adult life. Without this basic pattern of order, chaos results.

I experienced this myself when I moved out of my college dorm into a summer rental. I slept in, hung out with friends, and enjoyed my freedom. I ate at odd times, skipped some meals altogether, and snacked constantly on sweets. I thought I was having an ideal summer. Life was fun and exciting. Although my daily schedule was chaotic, it wasn't unnatural. Everyone I knew had a similarly unpredictable schedule. However, after a year and a half, I was a mess: lethargic, moody, and mentally unfocused. Chaos had resulted in the absence of order. Fortunately, I had the chance to go to a macrobiotic study house where I participated in the daily program and assisted in classes and meal preparation. Within a week, I noticed that my lethargy, mood swings, and cravings for sweets were disappearing. Eating healthy meals on a consistent schedule stopped the chaos and put me on the path to health.

Healthy foods and regularity go hand in hand. If you practice one without the other—such as eating healthy food at irregular times or eating unhealthy meals regularly—it isn't as beneficial. You need both healthy foods and healthy rhythm; together, they enable intuition to thrive.

Exercise 7: Create Order through a Meaningful Schedule

Consider your schedule to see how you manage your time. There are two parts: 1) Recognize your work and activity schedule (exercise 7-1); 2) Recognize your eating schedule (exercise 7-2).

Exercise 7-1: Life Template

The following template is a reflection of your daily routine, of what goes on in your life on a regular basis. Most people organize work, recreation, school, and other activities by the week. Write your activities for the next week in the blocks of time below. (If you have a different schedule, please draw a chart that reflects your situation. Whatever you do is perfect for you.)

	Sun	Mon	Tues	Wed	Thu	Fri	Sat
AM							
Noon							
Aft							
PM							

Now, note when you schedule things. When do you work? Do you work early? Night shift? Flexible schedule? Do you have regular exercise time? Take classes? Drive kids to school? Does your schedule change through the year or by the week?

Exercise 7-2: Menu Template

The "Menu Template" coordinates with the "Life Template" (above) in real life. We will use both in developing menus throughout this book.

The following template is one of scheduling rather than specific foods. Write in the blocks below the times of your meals in the next week. (Most people eat on a consistent schedule during the day, often on a weekly rhythm. If you have a different pattern, please draw a chart that reflects your meal times.)

	Sun	Mon	Tues	Wed	Thu	Fri	Sat
Breakfast							
Lunch							
Snack							
Dinner							

Now, notice the patterns of your meals:

1. When do you eat? Is the time consistent each day?

2. How many times do you eat? I like three meals with a snack in the afternoon. My husband likes four smaller meals. My kids like three meals and two snacks.

3. How do you prefer meals? Big, small, medium? When is your big meal of the day?

This template is a reflection of how you feed yourself. It is contingent on how you manage time and your personal strategy for determining menus. The purpose of this exercise is to reflect on the habits you already have and how you intuitively work with your life schedule in order to plan and eat meals.

Summary

A schedule with regular eating, sleeping, and work patterns creates a rhythm that establishes order and harmony. Order structures the framework in which to create and reclaim intuition.

Lesson 8

Water

Water provides life. There is a way to ingest it
to utilize and heighten intuition.

Everyone agrees—from yoga teachers to doctors to parents—water is vital to your health. Water is necessary for digestion, respiration, elimination, and circulation. It is present in all organs, tissues, and fluids in the body. Water keeps the brain functioning, the digestive juices flowing, and the energy system of the body electrified. Water affects metabolism, removes toxins, and enables nutrients to flow in and out of cells. Most diseases respond to water because water promotes healing.

Just like the "water planet" we live on, we have the same percentage of water. Both the earth and our bodies are about 75% water. With a percent this high, it is important to drink enough water and to know the best ways to obtain and consume it.

Your body uses a certain amount of water each day in normal processes. When there are additional stressors—such as disease, medications, strenuous exercise, dehydration, or even living in a dry climate—your body requires more water. Ideally, the proportion of fluids in your body is in balance so you function in the best way possible.

Thirst is the intuitive drive of your body to make you drink water. Your thirst mechanism ensures you don't become dehydrated and, for most people, it is automatic. However, many things affect your response to your thirst mechanism. Have you ever been thirsty but withheld drinking because you couldn't stop to go the bathroom in the next 30 minutes? Maybe you reached for a soda or coffee when thirsty—both beverages that are actually dehydrating—or eaten a snack rather than drink water. Maybe you were too busy to pause and take a drink of water. Maybe—like me—you once drank a big glass of water and felt waterlogged, so now you don't reach for big glasses of water.

If neglected, the thirst mechanism can die down. It is possible to lose awareness of thirst, drink too little water, and eventually become dehydrated. The author of *Your Body's Many Cries for Water*, Fereydoon Batmanghelidj, M.D, outlines the seriousness of a lack of water—from disease progression and aging to a slowing of metabolism and foggy thinking. His recommendation is to drink water not only to replenish the inner stores but also to maintain or reactivate the thirst mechanism.

Exercise 8: How to Drink Water

The objective of this exercise is to learn to consciously drink water, both to hydrate your body and to begin the process of reclaiming your innate thirst drive if it is missing or diminished. This technique enhances your health and utilizes your intuition.

Take one mouthful of water and hold it in your mouth. Swish the water through your teeth briefly and feel your saliva mingle with the water. Be conscious of the water as you swallow. Repeat with each mouthful. Some people call this method, "Chewing your water." This way of drinking has many benefits:

1. *Satisfies dry mouth.* Holding water in your mouth briefly before swallowing soothes and moistens your mouth cavity so you don't overdrink.

2. *Is gentle on the body.* Water enters your stomach in small amounts rather than a huge quantity. When you're really thirsty, instead of gulping down a large glass of water, slow down and drink the same quantity over a period of 15 to 30 minutes. Notice the difference.

3. *Regulates water intake immediately.* If eating a meal, drink water one mouthful at a time and mix with saliva. Some people advise against drinking with meals, especially a large amount of liquid at once. But, drinking one mouthful at a time especially in between bites of food will not dilute stomach fluids or cause the lower stomach sphincter to open as it does when a large quantity of water is drunk quickly.

4. *Regulates water intake throughout the day.* Sip water at regular intervals to stay hydrated. This adds moisture to your body in increments and maintains a constant level of fluid. Over time, your thirst mechanism will reactivate, and the habit of sipping water regularly will become automatic.

5. *Rejuvenates your body.* Water is needed for proper bodily functions; consciously sipping water throughout the day

contributes to a smooth metabolism. If you have health concerns, from major ones such as cancer to minor ones such as retaining water, this method of drinking replenishes the water in your body in small doses. If you are dehydrated or very thin, this method of drinking gradually adds fluid to your body.

6. *Can help you change.* Drinking sodas, high-fructose drinks, alcohol, or coffee can create a fluid imbalance and other problems. Do your best to replace them with pure water. If you are trying to lose weight, drink water before eating; you will feel satisfied with less food.

If you wish to increase your daily consumption of water, drink this way often, up to four times per hour on the first day. Pay attention to how you feel and whether it is agreeable. Every day, continue as is comfortable. It can take a month or longer to notice any differences. Some people report changes in skin, elimination, sleeping, and other functions.

Summary

Water is necessary for life, just like food, but there is a major difference. You can survive for a few weeks without food, but only a day or so without water. Make sure to drink pure water daily. The exercise presented will help you in many ways—from regularizing to increasing your water intake. Most of all, it will help reactivate your thirst mechanism and your intuition about water.

Lesson 9

Claims

Truth and claims are not the same thing. Decide the truth of claims for yourself; doing so empowers you to live your own truth.

Claims are everywhere! Doctors, politicians, teachers, parents, authors, and advertisers state *such and such* will help, insist that *such and such* is preferable, or proclaim that *such and such* is the best. How can a person determine the truth of such claims?

Truth is universal—true for everyone all the time. No one refutes it. For instance, everyone accepts the fact that humans need water for existence. Claims, on the other hand, are subjective. As concerns water, there are various claims about what kind of water to drink, how much to consume, and which filtration system to use, if any. Spring water, mountain water, filtered water, ionized water...so many types of water, so many claims.

In addition to claims about products, there are claims about experiences. My older brother played football in high school. One hot day after a strenuous practice, he guzzled cupfuls of ice water from the team's five-gallon water thermos. He developed severe stomach cramps. He claimed that icy cold water was a bad thing and that he would never drink it again after working so hard. He stressed that I should never do it either.

Some claims are relayed secondhand. A friend overheard a conversation between two adult swimmers. They were discussing hydration for swimmers and the fact that swimmers can dehydrate even though they are in water. The first swimmer maintained that sports drinks hydrate the cells. The other disagreed and said that boiled water helps the most. When I told this story to yet another friend, he commented that he had a similar experience. He boiled water, cooled it, and then drank it throughout the day. He felt the boiled water hydrated him and that his body absorbed the water better because he no longer had to use the bathroom in the middle of the night.

Many claims are made by advertisers. At a meeting I attended for a multilevel company promoting water filtration systems, the speaker said that during autopsies, coroners often find the internal organs dehydrated—sometimes even when the body has excess water weight. He claimed his product was superior to provide pure water to hydrate the body.

Claims are entertaining, often informative, and sometimes inspiring. The point in this lesson is not so much, "Are they true?" but rather, "How should I respond?"

How do you determine whether or not to believe a claim or act on it? While you need to consider the source and any personal expectations, it is important to become educated—to learn about the product and its value. Note whether the experience relayed appears to be boasting or has merit. It is truly worthwhile to learn how to discern when a claim is useful.

Education provides the information we need to understand and evaluate. Practice develops the awareness we need to make informed choices. A beginning step is to learn to analyze claims. Today, we practice with water.

Exercise 9: How to Verify Claims of Water

This exercise helps determine the validity of claims in regard to water. As in Exercise 8, take a drink of water and hold it in your mouth briefly, mingling it with saliva. Taste it. Savor it. Sense it for its flavor and the satisfaction it provides. Swallow and pay attention to how your stomach feels and whether or not it is agreeable. Just pay attention. If there is a particular claim around this water, consider whether you agree.

Repeat this exercise with a different water such as bottled instead of filtered, boiled instead of tap, or a second brand of bottled water. Taste the second type in the same manner as the first. Let the water mix with saliva and again determine the taste, satisfaction, and feel in the stomach. How do they compare? You can repeat this with as many types of water as you want, and especially when you are exposed to a claim about a specific water or filtration system.

While this exercise focuses on water, it can be used to validate other claims about foods and products.

Summary

In the journey of life, there are countless claims. You are exposed to them daily, as you will be for your entire life. My desire in this book is not to convince you to do what I do, but to help you develop your own intuition so you can determine for yourself. Recognize that there are claims around you all the time and that you can determine for yourself whether the claim is valid for you or not. No matter what the claim, the final assessment of the validity of the claim is your right, your responsibility, and within your power. This is exercising your intuition.

Lesson 10

Catalyst

Never underestimate life's experiences and never undermine your own path. The life you live is your own; no one else can live it for you. A catalyst is a signal to claim the health and happiness that is your intuitive right.

A catalyst provides a wake-up call that says it is time to take care of something; it is an event that causes a change. A catalyst is more than behavior modification, which is usually a minor adjustment that eases a specific situation. A catalyst, on the other hand, leads to a big change, a life-altering experience, a fork in the road of life where a person decides to take a turn or follow a new course.

Sometimes behavior modifications lead to catalysts or catalysts may initiate behavior modifications. Generally, the difference is an internal one—catalysts cause a change in attitude that transforms one's life.

When it happened to me, I didn't see it coming. I was addicted to cigarettes and marijuana as a teenager, and I smoked everyday. The incongruity is that I had seasonal hay fever with allergic reactions to pollens and molds, and had been taking allergy shots since childhood. Deep down, I knew that smoking made my allergies worse, but I insisted it helped me feel better as smoke literally dried my constant nasal drip. Besides, I didn't want to stop. Nor could I.

At 19, it occurred to me that I would eventually have to pay for my own medication, so I began to look for alternatives. I worked at a health food store (another irony: everyone who worked there smoked!) and heard lots of advice about allergy relief, such as taking thousands of milligrams of vitamin C, supplementing with bee pollen, eating miso, and drinking large quantities of water. No one suggested quitting smoking. One piece of advice made me scoff—try acupuncture. This was 1979; acupuncture was new to this country and practiced in the backs of offices; it was not recognized as legitimate. A month later, another person suggested it. Six months later, I took a chance and made an appointment.

When I went in for the first visit, the acupuncturist said, "You smoke pot, right?" I looked at the floor, shuffled my feet, and mumbled, "How do you know?" I wasn't high at that moment, and my clothing smelled fresh from riding my bike to the office. "I can tell by the way you walk," he said. He insisted that I quit and that he wouldn't do treatments if I smoked pot. "No," I responded. I wasn't going to stop. I turned to the door.

"Wait," he said. I turned and faced him. "Would you be willing to avoid pot for the rest of the day? I could give you a treatment today and you would get some benefit...." I thought about it and agreed. I could refrain from smoking for a few hours. I lay on the table, and he inserted needles in my fingers and toes. I breathed and relaxed for 20 minutes, wondering what my friends would think.

I arose as a new woman. I rode my bike the two miles home standing on the pedals, like a 4th grader in a race. I had energy and exuberance and couldn't wait to tell my roommate. I was clear-headed, happy, and felt full of life. Pot smoking had never left that kind of high.

The enthusiastic feeling passed the next day with the first puff of marijuana, but the memory was so wonderful that I decided to make another appointment. For this visit, I avoided pot for hours before the treatment. Again, it was energizing and again I raced home standing on the pedals of my bike.

This was a new kind of high, leaving me with a clear mind and eagerness to do things rather than feeling lethargic and unmotivated. I couldn't wait to have another treatment; so, I made another appointment. Yet, even with this drastic change of feeling, I couldn't abandon my habits or friends. I scheduled the treatment midweek so the weekend was free to party.

Over the next six weeks, I continued this pattern but gradually became aware of something—the pot high wasn't worth it. On the day of treatment, I felt clear and clean. I was more productive at work. On the days when I smoked, I was tired and made more mistakes. By the 7th week, I made a decision to expand the non-smoking days to 3 days. By the 12th week, I was ready to take a full week off pot. By the 16th week, I made the commitment to remain pot-free forever. Three months later, I quit tobacco and haven't smoked since. In 2010, I celebrated 30 years of being smoke-free!

Acupuncture was the catalyst that changed my life. It began as a wake-up call for remedial treatment of allergies and fear of medical bills. It culminated in freedom from addiction to tobacco and marijuana. I received a gift for life. At the time, I recognized it was a big change. Now I know it was an event that possibly saved my life. I could have headed down a completely different road.

It took time; it didn't happen overnight. The ability to compare the effects of acupuncture with the effects of marijuana was valuable. The acupuncturist's treatments helped my physical body regain balance so it could be free of addiction. As my body became healthier, my mind became stronger. I was able to be firm in the choice to be smoke-free, regardless of what my friends thought.

This was my wake-up call, my catalyst for change. I still get goose bumps thinking of it. It inspires me not only because of the difficulty of conquering addiction, but also because of the inner commitment I made to help myself.

The lessons for me are many and I still learn from this experience. I review this event and garner new insights. A catalyst is like this, offering help at the time, inspiration for the future, and encouragement over time.

Exercise 10: Recall a Catalyst

This is a reflective exercise—to examine a catalytic event in your own life. Think of a particular situation that you would characterize as a wake-up call or catalyst. Be easy and gentle in this evaluation. If this is a stressful remembrance, you may wish to seek qualified help to walk you through the details. It is also acceptable to choose a less stressful example.

Recollect the experience, recall your thinking, and state the positive benefit you received. Call up specifics. What happened? How did you react? What did you do? What was the immediate need? What were the long-lasting effects? Did anything change?

Remember your specific thoughts. Did you have ideas such as, "I must do thus and such or else this or that will happen?" Try to recall emotions too and any relevant feelings of joy, hope, fear, anxiety, etc. Again, be as gentle as possible with yourself.

Positive and negative thoughts, feelings, and actions precipitate change. Ideally, a positive attitude brings long-lasting change. Do your best to find a positive meaning in the experience. If the experience effected a permanent change for the better, you have a reason to celebrate.

Finish on a positive note. Remind yourself that you did something to help yourself, regardless of negative or positive impulse.

Know that you had strength and courage to see it through and that this power is within you, always available and always inspiring.

Summary
A catalyst signals a big event. It means more than a change in behavior. It is an intuitive sign from deep within yourself to activate your power.

Lesson 11

Habits

Use your habits as tools for enlightenment, not as a means to sink into routine and apathy.

Habits are universal. Many are beneficial such as brushing your teeth after eating. Others make life easier, such as driving a specific route to work that avoids traffic congestion.

Good habits focus on healthy actions. Parents and teachers strive to instill many good patterns in young children so they will carry them into adulthood. Some of my good habits that I taught to my kids are: washing hands after using the bathroom and removing muddy shoes before entering the house. You probably have similar habits you encourage.

While good habits are desired, bad habits are a part of life too. Like good habits, bad ones also develop over time, but usually without much awareness. Some are bothersome such as watching too much television, losing track of time, or leaving wet towels on furniture. Other bad habits such as smoking cigarettes, drinking excessive alcohol, or taking drugs can develop into addictions and require intervention and/or a strong will to break free.

Any habit can become routine and be done without thinking.

Often, this is not a problem; it is just an automatic reaction such as covering your mouth when you cough. Other habits such as poor posture can develop into problems like curvature of the spine. Some habits require thinking so a person remains focused; driving is a perfect example of a habit that requires attention to remain safe. Luckily, variations in traffic, weather, road conditions, and traffic lights help a person stay alert.

A simple change in routine increases your consciousness about routine activities and eases the boredom of repetitive chores. Thus, it is a good practice to intentionally vary routine habits in small ways. For example, shave each day starting at a different spot or vacuum the carpets beginning in a different room each time.

Exercise 11: Eat One Slice of Bread.

It is important to be aware of your habits during eating. Read the following directions, gather the materials, and allow uninterrupted time for this exercise.

Eat a slice of bread slowly and consciously and observe your habits. Do your best to obtain the healthiest whole grain bread available. If possible, avoid refined flours and, especially, refined sugar in the bread used for this exercise.

> ◊ *If you were at my house, I would give you a slice of whole grain naturally leavened bread made of whole grain flour, water, and sea salt.*

Do your best to practice each of the following nine steps as thoroughly as possible. Apply one step at a time. Don't jump ahead or combine steps until directed to do so.

> ◊ *If you were at my house, I would coach you through the steps one at a time.*

You may wish to do this exercise at some other time than meals. If at mealtime, practice this exercise first and then proceed with the rest of the meal. For optimal benefits, practice alone, unless your companions are also doing this exercise. Sit and be silent so you can be completely aware of what you are doing.

1. Use one slice of bread, toasted if desired. Eat it plain; don't spread anything on it. Divide it into nine bites. Eat the first piece normally—whatever "normally" means to you.

2. For the second bite, count how many times you chew it and consciously mix your saliva with the bread. Notice whether or not the taste of this bite is different from the first one.

3. For the third bite, repeat the counting and chewing; savor and enjoy the bread.

For the remaining steps, chew each bite as long as possible and count if desired.

4. For the fourth bite, notice how you are sitting. Be aware of the chair, the floor, and your posture, feet, and hands.

5. For the fifth bite, adopt a healthy posture, such as hands relaxed in lap, feet flat on the floor, spine straight, eyes closed, and breathing steady. Alter anything as necessary to be comfortable.

6. For the sixth bite, observe how you chew, whether slowly or quickly. Both ways have benefits.

7. For the seventh bite, change the speed. If you chewed slowly in step 6, quicken the pace. If you chewed rapidly, slow down. Notice any difference.

8. For the eighth bite, repeat the new speed you adopted in step 7. It is said that slow chewing is calming, and quick chewing is energizing. Do you find this to be true?

9. For the ninth and last bite, relax as you unify these practices of consciously mixing food with saliva, maintaining a healthy posture, and chewing at the speed of your choice. Breathe regularly, enjoy this last bite, and smile in appreciation for any new information gleaned from this practice.

Summary

Habits are powerful and worthwhile "tools" that help in all manner of circumstances. Use this practice of eating to raise your consciousness and to become aware of a new dimension of the art of eating. With any change in habit, intuition has a chance to grow.

Lesson 12

REVIEW: **Impetus to Change**

A change initiated from within is personal growth.

Change is an inevitable part of life. And, even though you know that change will happen, change can be scary for almost everyone. When changes occur, there can be an upheaval—an unsettling time when normal things come undone. Particularly when change is caused by outside influences, it can seem an imposition such as when one person insists that you do something differently. Yet, change initiated from within can be a lifesaver such as when a catalyst motivates a change that has a long-term benefit. These types of changes can spark a lot of growth and significantly raise your consciousness.

The five lessons in Unit 2 are about change, covering aspects of why to change and how to embrace change. The exercises present ways to help you initiate change in your life. Together, the lessons and exercises relate to the theme presented at the beginning of the unit: What you know can be used as a springboard for change. You start where you are and move forward, changing as needed to help yourself now and in the future. In the process, you trust that you are benefiting from the change.

Here are summaries of the five lessons in Unit 2:

Lesson 7: Rhythm. Rhythm creates order, which in turn helps you reclaim intuition.

Lesson 8: Water. Water is best drunk intuitively, one sip at a time.

Lesson 9: Claims. Claims can be true or false and need to be evaluated for yourself using your intuitive power of integrity.

Lesson 10: Catalyst. Some events are so powerful that they dictate an outward change of behavior and are an intuitive message to take care of yourself.

Lesson 11: Habits. Habits are tools we can use to foster intuitive awareness.

These five lessons drive home another point: How to listen and act on internal wisdom. Our bodies convey a lot of information. If we "tune in," we can tap into our natural wisdom. Often, natural wisdom communicates through an inner voice. Have you ever thought or said to yourself, "I really shouldn't have this?" or "I really should do such and such?" Your internal voice speaks a lot and its messages are often preceded by the words *should* or *shouldn't*.

Our inner voice often signals that there needs to be a change right now. For example, if you feel you shouldn't be eating something or doing something, pay attention. Likewise, if you feel you should be eating or doing something, pay attention.

These signals are important. Sometimes they are a call for help, especially if there is an addiction. Other times, they are a prompt to do something differently. The deeper meaning is that these signals are a desire for change.

Exercise 12: Do I Really Want to Eat This?

The exercise today is a reflective one to practice at various eating times to sharpen your internal response system. At least three separate times during the day, with three different foods, ask yourself, "Do I really want to eat this?" Notice your reaction. There is no right or wrong answer here, and this is not a test of willpower or an exercise in growth. It is practice in noticing your internal awareness.

This exercise can help you stop eating when full or identify times when it is okay to indulge. For instance, there are times when I really want chocolate; other times not. Sometimes I have heard myself say "Stop" after one cookie. Sometimes I'm at a potluck and really don't want to eat certain dishes.

Summary

Change is not to be feared, especially when it it driven by internal signals. Learn to pay attention to these messages and to trust them. This is using your intuition.

The Good Life

Concentrate on the beauty you want in your life
and learn how to increase it.

Everyone wants a good life of health, happiness, and a promising future. Having hope that this is possible can be challenging in today's world. In this unit, you'll learn about gaining a perspective that interprets events or circumstances from a positive point of view. You'll learn to be optimistic.

Keyword: Optimism

The main objective for this unit is learning to cultivate or enhance optimism. Optimism is based on awareness, and awareness is based on reality, relevancy, and potential, i.e., where you are at the moment, what is important to you, and what you desire. Your present life is valuable—where you are is a culmination of all you have experienced; it is a beautiful place. Use your awareness of all aspects of your life to help you set a direction for the future. This engages your intuition, which will help you live the life you want.

Food: Limited Fasting

Food and your relationship to food are central in the lessons of Unit 3. In Lesson 16, there is a limited fast of brown rice and steamed vegetables. In the days before the fast, spend time cooking healthy foods and eating meals consciously and with awareness.

Exercise: Prepare for Fast

Plan your time and determine your meals to coordinate with the lessons. Do this exercise before starting lesson 13:

1. Use the *Life Template* from Lesson 7 to decide which day to fast. This practical planning aligns the lessons with your life.

2. Use the *Menu Template* from Lesson 7 to outline meals that will work for you. This is planning for your comfort.

3. Plan menus for the meals before the fast to be healthy— whatever that means to you—and *realistic*—according to your available time and preferences. Lesson 15 encourages inclusion of a grain of your ancestors for one of the meals.

4. Lesson 16 is the day of the fast. Brown rice and steamed vegetables are suggested for all meals. Do your best to plan accordingly.

5. Lesson 17 is the day after the fast. Include more protein that day and a good source of fat to help avoid cravings, binges, or out-of-control eating. Consume sensible portions.

6. Lesson 18 is the second day after the fast. Continue to eat sensible portions of quality ingredients.

Note: In preparing for the fast, use common sense about your ability to do this. If you have health concerns or any question as to the appropriateness of fasting, discuss the pros and cons with your health care practitioner. In addition, be gentle with yourself in order to avoid any extremes. It is important to transition in and out of a fast consciously.

Resources: Appendix 3

◊ *Addictions*
◊ *Cravings*
◊ *Intuition about Salt and Spices*
◊ *Intuition about Oils*

Getting Started: Lessons 13 to 18

In lessons 13 to 18, you discover ways to make your life better. You acknowledge your present level of health and comfort. You learn how your past contributes to your strengths. You plan for the future by setting goals. All of these activities cultivate your optimism and reinforce your belief that life is good.

Lesson 13

Considerations

Consider the possibility that life is large,
and there is much potential.

Consider the big (future) picture—what you want overall—and images will expand to fill your mind with tremendous possibilities. Consider the little (immediate) picture—what you want to be different now—and images will arrive of how to make your present life better.

It is fantastic to consider both big pictures and little pictures. In this lesson, you consider your little picture (your present) in order to understand how to affect your big picture (your future). Both pictures are important; they affect each other. For today and the next few lessons, we will talk of the little picture, so that by the review lesson at the end of this unit, we will be ready to talk about the big picture.

In any self-awareness or self-improvement program, there are three general steps:

1. *Evaluation*: Consider the situation. Ask who, what, when, where, why, and how. Who is involved? What is the situation? When did it happen? Why is this important? How do I address this situation?

2. *Education*: Gather information, consult books or people for advice, and educate yourself about the possibilities. Ask questions. What do I need to know? What should I do and how will I do it? Will such and such help? When or where do I go? Who can I ask for help?

3. *Action*: Act on what you learned in step two. Sometimes action requires tremendous courage; sometimes it requires patience. Above all else, actions that arise from deep personal convictions provide the greatest benefits—long lasting benefits that affect the big picture.

It is possible to act blindly, to approach life's activities and challenges without any plan or intention; this is groping in the dark. To be in control and have power, one must "turn on the light!" This means taking the necessary steps to *evaluate, educate,* and *act*. These three steps are important in any activity related to change, whether it is diet, career, or relationship.

Exercise 13: Consider Your Diet at Various Times in Your Life

Evaluate your past diet and routines to gain information about your upbringing and your strength of character. Review the specific foods, habits, and attitudes about food that have sustained you thus far in your life. You often remember certain foods and the specific environments that shaped your relationship to those foods as well as food in general. Positive attitudes contribute to intuition; do your best to recall positive influences related to consuming food.

Write down answers to the following questions about what you ate and your overall feelings surrounding food at different times in your life. This is meant to be a positive activity; if memories arise that are stressful, you can focus on comfortable associations.

Infancy: Primary Nourishment
◊ What did you eat when you were a baby?
◊ Were you breast- or bottle-fed?

◊ What were comfort foods?

◊ What is something positive you received from your mother or caretaker regarding your original source of nourishment?

Childhood: Orderliness.

◊ What did you eat as a young child once you could feed yourself?

◊ Did you have rhythms in your food habits?

◊ What were foods you usually ate at breakfast, lunch, dinner, and snack times?

◊ What is something positive you received from your family and/or siblings about regularity and orderliness?

School age: Social influences.

◊ What did you eat at school, and especially around friends?

◊ Did your peers influence your food choices?

◊ What were foods you enjoyed at social gatherings?

◊ What is something positive you received from your friends about camaraderie and food?

Young adulthood: Independence.

◊ What foods did you eat during the first years when you were on your own and began to choose your own meals?

◊ Did you have control of your consumption?

◊ What is something positive you accomplished as you began your life apart from your parents?

Adulthood to present: Establishment of habit.

◊ What foods have you usually eaten since becoming independent?

◊ Have you experimented with various diets?

◊ What are your customary habits of eating: eating take-out or at restaurants, consuming fast food, cooking for yourself, giving dinner parties?

◊ What is something positive you built through the years in nourishing yourself?

Summary

Food has nourished you all your life—during infancy, school years, and adulthood. It fed your body as you grew and influenced your feelings as you interacted with others. No matter the experience, good or bad, food enabled you to live and continue to grow each day. It is the foundation for your body, mind, and spirit; it is a key source of intuition.

Lesson 14

Possibility

Admire the beauty and truth of your body.

Your body is marvelous! If you stop and consider how it operates, you realize it is a miracle. When you acknowledge your body's internal wisdom, you can't help but appreciate and admire its beauty.

However—and this is a big however—this beauty is usually hidden. Most people have pain somewhere: pain that hides the beauty; pain that hides the marvel; pain that hides the internal wisdom. Pain is so common that everyone thinks it is normal and natural. Have you ever considered the possibility that pain has a different meaning?

At its most basic level, pain is an intuitive message that an area of the body needs attention. It is your body's way of telling you— loud and clear—"Pay attention right here...right now!" Discomfort, restlessness, and unease are other symptoms that communicate the same thing...as does "dis-ease."

Reactions to symptoms vary. One response is denial; people ignore signs of pain and areas of distress. Fear is another reaction; pain may indicate serious disease or degeneration. Optimally, pain is a catalyst that initiates a search for healing.

Exercise 14: Consider Twelve Areas of the Body

This exercise a dual purpose: 1) To appreciate your body and all it does; 2) To see beyond pain to the deeper intuitive message. It concentrates on your body.

There are twelve body systems with related organs, basic functions, and a general meaning of pain within each. This is not a medical exercise; rather, it is simply a suggestion of the possible intuitive messages connected to pain.

You will need privacy and ample time to do this exercise. Place your hand over each of the approximate areas named below in succession. Notice whether you have any pain or discomfort in that area. Pause with each step and acknowledge that your body usually continues to function despite discomfort. Even with pain, your body is dependable. How amazing is that?

System One: Cardiovascular—Open to Life

The heart, blood vessels, and blood constitute the cardiovascular system. The heart circulates blood throughout your body, ceaselessly carrying oxygen and nutrients to your cells. Place one hand over your heart and notice your heartbeat. Appreciate your heart and blood for pulsating life. If you have pain or diagnosed disease, consider (the possible message of) how to become more open to life, to oxygen, and to love.

System Two: Urinary—Fullness of Life

The urinary system includes kidneys, ureters, and bladder. The kidneys help regulate water in the body and work nonstop in maintaining homeostasis, that is, a state of balance. Place your hands over your kidneys (lower middle back) and appreciate your kidneys for monitoring the 70% of your body that is water. If you have kidney problems, consider (the possible message of) how you hold and encompass the fullness of life.

System Three: Respiratory—Give and Take

Lungs, bronchi, and nasal passages comprise the respiratory system. The lungs inhale oxygen and exhale carbon dioxide. Place your hands over your lungs, breathe deeply, and appreciate your lungs for their capacity to process air. If you have any pain or difficulty in breathing, consider (the possible message of) how to increase equality and tolerance in areas of give and take in your life.

System Four: Defense—Caring for Self

The skin and immune system are two parts of your defense system. The skin is like a shield that protects the body from outside influences. The skin grows with age, stretches with movement, breathes and interacts with the environment when sweating. It is also your physical presence in the world. Place one hand over your other hand and notice your skin. Appreciate it for its function and appearance. Disease or pain anywhere in or on the skin is related to boundaries. Consider (the possible message of) how you stand up for yourself and take care of yourself, from the outside in.

The immune system is your internal defense system. It is an integrated support system of white blood cells, endocrine system glands, and liver and pancreas. The immune system, like the skin, interacts with all systems of the body. Place one hand over your liver and appreciate your immune system for how it works with everything else in your body. If you have pain anywhere in your body, it involves your immune system. Consider (the possible message of) how you take care of yourself, from the inside out.

System Five: Digestive—Ingest and Digest

The digestive tract consists of the mouth to stomach to intestines with input from liver, pancreas, and gall bladder. The digestive tract works in stages throughout the day as it breaks down and assimilates food. Place your hands over your stomach and appreciate your digestive system for delivering nutrition to your body. If you have any pain or discomfort, consider (the possible message of) how you ingest and digest the richness of life.

System Six: Nervous—Cognitive Ability and Communication

Your brain, spinal cord, nerves, and sensory receptors constitute your nervous system. The brain is the control network of your body, enabling you to think, comprehend, remember, and feel. The nervous system coordinates all areas of your body. Place your hands on your head; appreciate your brain for how intelligent it is and your nervous system for connecting your entire body. If you have pain in your brain or nerve pain, consider (the possible message of) how smart you are. Recognize that your internal communication system is telling you about areas that need help.

System Seven: Lymphatic—Deal with Waste

This system includes your lymph nodes, tonsils, and spleen. The lymph system filters blood, removes excess byproducts, and helps avoid toxicity. The health of the kidneys and liver affect the lymphatic system as each organ filters blood and removes toxins. Place your hands over your tonsils in your neck or over your lymph nodes in your armpit; appreciate your body for being able to filter and discharge impurities. If you have pain in these areas, consider (the possible message of) how to lighten your load.

System Eight: Endocrine—Small Things Have Power

Your endocrine system is composed of glands: pituitary, pineal, thyroid, parathyroid, thymus, pancreas, adrenals, ovaries (females), and testes (male). Glands provide hormones to control bodily functions, such as growth, metabolism, digestion, and reproduction. Gently place your hand over your thyroid at the front of your throat; appreciate your glands for their presence in your body. If you have pain, sluggishness, or are diagnosed with a disease in any of these areas, consider (the possible message of) how to actualize your full potential.

System Nine: Reproductive—Contributions

Our reproductive systems differ by gender: *Female*: fallopian tubes, uterus, vagina, and ovaries. *Male*: penis and testes. The reproductive system produces offspring. Place hands over lower abdomen (women) or over scrotum (men) and appreciate the fact that your body can create life. If you have pain or diagnosed disease in these areas, consider (the possible message of) how you are a unique person and have things that you contribute.

System Ten: Skeletal—Foundation

Your bones are the frame of your body, which supports all your muscles and organs. Bones store calcium, and bone marrow produces red blood cells. Place one hand over the other wrist and notice your bones. Appreciate your bones for physical strength, ability to hold you up and move you around, and capacity to manufacture blood. If you have pain in bones, consider (the possible message of) how to strengthen your foundation of power.

System Eleven: Muscular—Action and Rest

Muscles cover the entire body, provide flesh, and store fat, water, minerals, and vitamins. Place one hand over the biceps of the opposite arm and appreciate how they flex and relax. If you have pain in muscles, consider (the possible message of) how to balance action with adequate recuperation.

System Twelve: Energy—Soul

Your body's energy system of chakras and soul or spirit contains your life force. Place hands over the center of your being, wherever you consider this center to be and appreciate your overall physical energy. Appreciate the fact that you were once a child with a joy for living and that you still possess this capacity as an adult. If you have soul pain, which is difficult to describe other than uneasiness or a general feeling of "I need something else," consider (the possible message of) how to manifest your greatest capacity and recognize you have a special existence.

Summary

Your body is designed to do certain jobs, and it strives to function despite disease and pain. Honor these qualities. Recognize the natural power of your body. Pain is more than just discomfort; it is a signal from the innate wisdom of your body. Let pain be a guide—not a dictator—and a helpful reminder of your intuitive ability.

Lesson 15

Ancestors

Be aware of your heritage; it lives within you. The grain of your ancestors nourishes you.

Food keeps history alive. Have you ever eaten dishes that your grandparents ate? Or shared a favorite recipe with your kids or grandkids? Food spans generations—it binds families and constitutes cultures.

Usually when you go to a doctor or health practitioner, you provide your health history and list diseases of immediate family members. This information gives a glimpse of your genetic makeup and any predisposition toward disease. But your ancestors gave you more than DNA. If you have done a genealogical search, you may have discovered an ancestor who fought in a war, moved a great distance, or was famous. In uncovering your ancestral history, you may find traits and events that influence your own attitudes and character.

Uncovering your food history can be as fascinating. Food has an important relationship to heritage—both genetic and cultural. It determines health, affects attitudes, and forms the base of society. Think back to the agricultural revolution when the cultivation of crops became a turning point for humankind. Recorded history begins with hunter-gatherer societies that evolved into tribal societies that evolved into civilizations. Tools, governments, crafts, and foods developed as societies evolved. People cultivated, planted, and harvested crops to ensure surplus, and agriculture boomed.

The history of civilization parallels the cultivation of grains. Barley was one of the first grains cultivated in the Middle East—the area of the Fertile Crescent. Rice grew in India and China. Barley and oats grew in Europe. Corn and quinoa grew in the Americas.

Grains had a prominent place in each culture. People developed rituals for planting seeds and celebrating the harvest. They believed their gods and goddesses gave grains as gifts. Egyptian culture elevated grains to such a high place of honor that they placed kernels of grains in the graves of the Pharaohs.

Over time, grains continued to be the foundation of the food supply. When people migrated, they carried their seeds and adapted their grains to the new place. Different varieties developed; new foods and beverages appeared. It continues today—grains continue to be resettled as in the case of quinoa, a grain from the Peruvian Incas now grown in the United States. Grains are also hybridized, genetically modified, and refined… sometimes to their detriment. This is the case with high fructose corn syrup, a product of corn that is now linked to many health problems.

Eating grain in a whole, unprocessed form provides many benefits. It supports health and establishes a base for meal planning. (We'll cover this topic in depth throughout this book.) For today, the idea is to understand your personal link to your past—through grains.

Everyone has this link. Most people descended from civilizations that depended on grains for nourishment. Today, grains are consumed universally. Even though there are still tribes who hunt and gather and nomads who migrate to graze livestock, the majority of people today depend on cultivated food, especially grain. Rice feeds people in India, China, and Japan and throughout the Eastern World. Bread accompanies meals for people in Europe. Corn is common in South and Central America. Grains are so accepted that whenever there is famine or drought, relief organizations ship grain to the population in need. Universally, grain has passed from generation to generation, just like genetics and DNA. When you eat your ancestral grain, you tap into this history.

Exercise 15: Consume Grain of Ancestors

Today, the exercise is one of perceiving your inheritance from another perspective and connecting with your lineage at mealtime.

Consider your personal ancestry and find out which grains were common. You don't need to return to antiquity; backtrack to what your parents, grandparents, and great-grandparents ate. Chances are you will find that they consumed grain they grew themselves, or if they weren't farmers, grain that was cultivated nearby. It may not have been the majority of the meal, but it had a place on the table, probably every day. Some examples are: oats, rye, barley, or wheat for Northern Europe and Scandinavia; corn for Native Americans; rice for Japan, China, and India; millet, sorghum, and teff for Africa. Ireland had barley before potatoes. Europe had barley and rye before wheat. The foods made from grains are many: bread, pasta, tortillas, porridge, and crackers.

Prepare the food you select based on your ancestry and think of how this grain nourished your ancestors. As you eat it, chew it well.

Summary

The foods of your ancestors nourished them as your genetic line passed from generation to generation. When you consume these foods, you strengthen the knowledge that is present in the depths of your cells and reinforces intuitive memory of your heritage.

Lesson 16

Fasting

Pause. Think. Simplify.

Fasting is a respite from food and from everyday life. Today's fast provides a pause from ordinary activities. There are many positive benefits. Fasting prepares you physically, mentally, and spiritually for change and growth. Used carefully and judiciously and, if needed, under supervision, fasts are safe and healthy. Anyone in good health can fast. People who are frail, elderly, or in a state of disease should proceed carefully and fast only in the sense of avoiding foods that contain refined sugar, are overly processed, or contain dyes and additives. Anyone in this condition should always consume nutritionally sound and well-balanced meals. If you have any question about whether or not fasting is appropriate for your state of health, consult your health practitioner. Also, please do not enforce a fast on a child or infant. Children need adequate calories and a wealth of nutrition. If you need to address a child's nutritional intake for health reasons, consult a doctor or nutritionist.

Fasting is used in many disciplines and diets because it can restore and revitalize. There are many types of fasts, such as: a total fast from all food and drink; a mono fast of water, juice, grapefruit, brown rice, or other solo food; a religious fast during a holiday such as avoiding meat for Lent or fasting all day for Ramadan; or a limited fast. Limited fasts have two elements: specific reductions and specific inclusions. Reduction can be either avoidance of certain items or decrease in quantity; inclusion is to consume certain items. Your limited fast today includes brown rice and vegetables and as much quantity as is comfortable. It is exclusive in that only these foods are used, although which vegetables to eat is up to you.

Fasting offers a chance to spend time in review. Many people fast for spiritual benefit. If you fast regularly or even only once, you may be familiar with the clarity of mind that results. If you have never intentionally fasted, think of a time, such as when you were ill, when you ate selectively or very small portions. I have found that I am much more particular about what I eat when I am sick.

Allow time to take it easy during your day of fast. Plan activities that are supportive of fasting and, if necessary, postpone the fast until the day is favorable. Many people fast on weekends because they don't work on Saturday and have Sunday to transition back to their regular routine.

This exercise has two parts: the fast itself and a time to reflect on your state of health using George Ohsawa's *Seven Conditions of Health*.

Exercise 16-1: Fast

Eat three meals today—one in the morning, one at noon, one in the evening. If the times don't coincide with morning or noon, space your meals throughout the day so there are a few hours between meals. You can drink small amounts of water at any time; take one sip at a time and swish the water with your saliva as practiced in Lesson 8. Don't gulp water or drink large quantities at one time.

For your meals, boil brown rice and steam any fresh vegetables you desire. You can cook once for all meals or cook each meal separately. You may use sea salt in cooking the brown rice, but avoid adding salt at the table. In addition, avoid soy sauce, miso, oil, nuts, protein foods, or any seasonings. If you are taking medications, consult your doctor before doing this limited fast.

At your meals, eat comfortable quantities. Chew each mouthful well. This will help saliva mingle with all your food and help you feel satisfied.

While you are fasting, think of how you/your body are getting a day of rest with brown rice and vegetables. If you experience any feelings of deprivation, remind yourself that this is only one day of fasting. Do your best to calm yourself. Drink some water and relax. If you have cravings, read the appendix on *Cravings and Addictions*.

Exercise 16-2: *Seven Conditions of Health, 1 to 3*

George Ohsawa was a Japanese philosopher who is generally considered the founder of modern macrobiotics, a discipline devoted to raising consciousness through integration of body, mind, and spirit. He emphasized healing the body through a wholesome diet, educating the mind through learning about dialectics, and integrating the spirit through connecting with the universe. His ideas, many of which are included in this course, come from a list titled *The Seven Conditions of Health*. Ohsawa felt that these conditions indicate a person's vitality. The first three relate to physical health, the fourth through sixth relate to the mind, and the seventh relates to spirit. To determine your status for each condition, answer the question presented in each.

1: Adequate Energy—No Fatigue

This condition refers to having enough stamina to do what is desired. A person with no fatigue is not too tired for physical work nor exhausted from the stresses of life.

◊ Do you have more than enough energy to do what you want?

2: Good Appetite

This condition refers to the ability to eat any food, simple or gourmet, and to be satisfied with both simplicity and complexity. Enjoyment comes from gratitude for the gift of life that food brings as well as gratitude for the person(s) who provided the food.

◊ Do you like simple food as well as gourmet food?

3: Restful Sleep

This condition is about rejuvenation from sleep. The hours are not as important as the restfulness.

◊ Do you fall asleep soon after lying down, sleep without disturbing dreams, and wake up feeling refreshed?

Evaluate your own state in these areas. Be gentle with yourself if you feel you rate low; you can improve these conditions over time. Today as you fast, pay attention to these areas and determine whether there is any difference from your regular feeling.

Summary

Fasting is a wonderful way to help refine your ability to taste, develop your intuition, and appreciate food. Many great teachers and spiritual leaders encourage fasting and prayer as a way to heal and a way to reach truth. Have a great day!

Lesson 17

Appetite

It is possible to return appetite to a desire for nourishment—to have an appetite for foods that sustain, enliven, and promote vitality.

How was your limited fast yesterday? Did you enjoy your respite? Did you savor your meals? Are you prepared for today?

Today's lesson is about having an appetite for healthy foods and regaining it if lost. This is not as hard as it sounds. Once you revive your appetite for healthy foods, you'll always remember how—hopefully you had a chance during the fast. Consciously choosing certain foods and consciously chewing them creates a change in your approach to food.

Your relationship to food is the secret. Appetite and hunger are words that describe our relationship to food. We often think they mean the same thing, but this is not the case as discussed previously. Hunger is for sustenance. Appetite is for taste. What is the difference? Hunger is general—we seek calories to survive. Appetite is selective—we seek flavors to satisfy.

Think of how we evolved in our life. As babies, we had hunger without selectiveness. We ate to live and didn't refuse any food. As we grew, we developed appetites for specific things. Even so, our appetites were simpler than they are now that we are adults.

Children want plain or unadorned food such as carrot sticks rather than mixed vegetables or simple pasta rather than a casserole. As a person ages, their preferences develop for specific attributes of food. Sometimes it's for sustenance; more often it is for taste or flavor. Adults want food that is pleasurable more than food that merely satisfies hunger. A slice of bread nourishes, yet the average adult considers it bland and puts something on it to enhance the taste.

Appetite is affected by other things, too. Flavor enhancers such as MSG, natural flavorings, and excess salt mask the original taste of food. Sometimes children won't drink juice after drinking a fruit-type drink with high-fructose corn syrup and flavor enhancers. Advertising warps perceptions about products by linking them with fun and sex or suggesting that people who eat truly healthy food are unpopular.

Another influence that taints appetite is addiction. Addiction to foods is prevalent in our culture, and many people can't get through the day without coffee, sugared foods, junk foods, or chocolate. It can be difficult to discern whether you are truly hungry or merely responding to an addiction. Breaking an addiction is one of the most powerful acts you can do for yourself. Although this lesson is not focused on the specifics of addictions, *Appendix 3* offers guidelines on how to address them.

For today, consider the idea that it is possible to have an appetite for foods that are wholesome. The hunger you had as a baby for pure food still resides within you. You can revive it and regain your appetite for wholesome and nourishing food.

I witnessed this in myself. I have been pregnant 5 times and, with each pregnancy, I tried to eat carefully. With the first and second pregnancies, I craved snacks and used willpower to stop eating excess chips and cookies (tried to, anyway). By the fourth and fifth pregnancies, the cravings changed—I longed for healthy food. I devoured cooked greens with umeboshi plum (Japanese salt plum)—a wonderful combination to obtain calcium from green vegetables. I wanted olive oil on salads, sea vegetables for minerals, beans and fish for protein, rather than chips, dairy foods, or salty snacks.

Never before or after have I sought such healthy food or had such repulsion for junk food. I still prefer this way of eating, even if not as strictly. The change in my appetite is permanent. Other people have said their desires for soft drinks, doughnuts, coffee, chocolate, and other foods have changed too.

Appetite for foods that nourish can be cultivated and achieved. This ability is possible because, deep down, everyone has the desire to live well. Appetite for nourishing food is your birthright to satisfy your hunger. It is possible to reclaim this birthright and experience rejuvenation. There are two steps to claiming this for yourself: 1) Select foods that are nourishing; and 2) Avoid foods that mask your true appetite.

Exercise 17-1: Break the Fast

The exercise today has two parts: 1) Break the fast of yesterday; 2) Eat sensible meals and comfortable portions all day. Specifically, eat nourishing healthy food such as brown rice and vegetables. Add a protein source such as beans, fish, or chicken. Use oils on salad or in vegetable dishes; include nuts, seeds, and fruit as desired.

To retrain your appetite, I suggest three actions:

◊ *Omit forever*: Items with food colorings, additives, artificial sweeteners, and high-fructose corn syrup.

◊ *Avoid for the duration of this course*: Items with white refined flour, white refined sugar, hydrogenated oils and trans fats, and commercial (not organic) dairy products and meat.

◊ *Be selective about*: Items that are potentially addictive, specifically the big three—white refined sugar, caffeine, and chocolate. In all cases, choose the best quality foods you can find.

Exercise 17-2: *Seven Conditions of Health, 4 to 7*

Consider the last four items from George Ohsawa's list of *The Seven Conditions of Health*. Items four, five, and six are qualities of the mind; item seven is a quality of the spirit.

4: Accurate Memory

This condition describes the ability that a person has to recall details, whether of people or events, past or present. A person does not deny or repress information but seeks to remember with honesty and kindness for all parties involved. This condition is related to thoughts.

◊ Can you remember names, places, and events, both short-term and long-term, as well as you always have?

5: Humor

This condition is one of enjoyment. A person embraces the ups and downs of life with steadfastness, facing challenges with courage and pleasantries with ease. This condition is related to emotions.

◊ Can you accept with gratitude both the good times and the bad times?

6: Clarity

This condition is one of thinking and acting appropriately. A person makes decisions without compromises, acts without harm, and responds without emotional outbursts. This condition is related to ethics: right actions and right thinking.

◊ Can you make a decision quickly and fairly for all involved and affected?

7: Mood of Justice—No Arrogance

This condition is one of appreciation for all that life has to offer. A person accepts life as it happens. There is no blame when things go wrong and no conceit when things go right. There is confidence in the order of the world and humility for one's personal contribution.

◊ Do you believe that everyone and everything is of value?

Summary

The conditions of health reflect basic life functions and the ideal state. While they all influence each other, good appetite (2) is a direct way to change the other conditions. Food affects energy (1), sleep (3), thoughts (4), emotions (5), ethics (6), and peacefulness (7).

We began this course with Exercise 1, eating one bite of food and appreciating all it has to offer. The fast yesterday was a pause from everyday experiences to appreciate simple food. I hope these exercises will help you have an appetite and hunger for nourishment—an act of fostering and strengthening intuition.

Lesson 18

REVIEW: The Good Life

It is possible to hope for a brighter future—one full of meaning, of joy, of life. Let your hopes be practical so you can manifest your dreams. Hope for appropriate things and be willing to do your part. Hope and responsibility go hand in hand.

Everyone wants a good life; everyone wants health and happiness. The theme of this unit is to discover ways to achieve those goals and make your life better. The lessons in this unit developed this theme by looking at the past and evaluating the present in order to prepare you for the lesson of planning for the future. Here are summaries of this unit's lessons:

Lesson 13: Considerations. Consider your past upbringing, specifically your diet and food habits, as the foundation for your intuition.

Lesson 14: Possibility. Consider your present situation, specifically the health of your body, and the possibility of translating any pain into intuitive awareness.

Lesson 15: Ancestors. Consider your past influences, specifically ancestors, and the foods that gave them strength.

Lesson 16: Fast. Pause from everyday routine and spend a day in the present moment.

Lesson 17: Appetite. Reintroduce your everyday routine and enjoy another day in the present moment.

Lesson 18 recaps these lessons and answers the question, "What would you change to make your life better?" You can also think of a related question, "What do you hope for?"

We all hope for things—health, peace, happy relationships, a fulfilling career. The secret is how to make our hopes come true.

Have you ever had a great vacation? Think for a minute of how you planned it such as booking a flight or obtaining a passport. When you dream of an ideal holiday, you plan before you step out of the door. The journey of your life is no different. Hope for things and then plan accordingly so that they occur.

It is important to build hopes on reasonable prospects. Hoping for sunshine in the middle of night is futile; build hope on things that are attainable. Some people hope that things will be different or that other people will do certain things. For highest benefit, put your hope in the things you have the most power over—the things you can do yourself rather than wishful thinking or promises from others. Hope for a brighter future and work to establish it. Hope for better health and align eating habits and lifestyle to reach this goal.

The exercise today elaborates on how to do so. There are three parts: past, present, and future. Read all three parts and then proceed through them one after the other.

Exercise 18-1: Setting Goals, Part 1—Past

This part of the exercise reviews the past—specifically ideas from the first 17 lessons in the course, as annotated in the following table that contains ideas about your relationship to food. Scan the list and determine how you have incorporated the behaviors, attitudes, and information. You might reread the lessons if you want to emphasize any of them in more detail. There is no need to strive for perfection: merely consider what you would like to address, if anything. This step prepares you for Part 2 of this exercise.

Behaviors (Lesson #)	Attitudes (Lesson #)	Information (Lesson #)
Chew food (1,2,3,4,5,6,11)	Decide for yourself (9)	Remove food clutter: Unit 1
Sit for meals (4,5,6)	Look for positive in situations (10,12,13,14,15)	Identify 12 areas of body and pain (14)
Say grace (4)	Review attitudes from upbringing (13)	Read about cravings and addictions (Appendix 3)
Avoid gulping water (8)		Create order today (7)
Avoid junk food (16,17)		Note conditions of health (16,17)
Eat wholesome foods every day: Units 1,2,3		Read about intuition about shopping and food groups (Appendices 1,2,3)

Exercise18-2: Setting Goals, Part 2—Present

The second part of this exercise focuses on the present—specifically what you need now. In this part, you identify your overall goal. Because this course is about food, your relationship to it, and the link to intuition, think of how you want the relationship to help you achieve your goal. Perhaps you need to change a behavior or diminish pain. Most people want health, happiness, and satisfaction; therefore, assume these are part of your goal—not your overall goal. Identify a specific goal that is necessary now. It may be tempting to think food is your goal. Again, it is better to think of food as the support for the things you want rather than as the goal in itself.

For myself, I have set the following overall goals at various times in my life:

"I want to have more energy to get my work done."
"I want to be healthy to keep up with my boys."
"I want my intuition to flourish."

These statements summarized my goals at a high level. For you, I recommend that you first identify your goal and write the following specifics for accomplishing a goal, reflected in the acronym SMART (Specific, Measurable, Attainable, Relevant, Time-based).

1. Specific
   a. What do you want to accomplish?
   b. Why do you want this goal? (Specific reasons, purpose, or benefits of accomplishing the goal.)
   c. Who is involved in reaching the goal?
   d. Where will work toward the goal occur?
   e. Which requirements and constraints exist?
   f. Write down this goal and the following attributes for achieving your goal.

2. Measurable
   a. What are your concrete criteria for measuring progress?
   b. How will you know when you have achieved your goal?

3. Attainable
   a. Is your goal realistic?

b. Do you have the necessary attitude, abilities, skills, and desire to reach this goal?

4. Relevant

a. Does this goal seem worthwhile? Does it reflect your innermost desires?
b. Is this the right time for you to work toward this goal?
c. Does this goal match your other efforts/wants at this time?
d. Is this goal consistent with your current perspective? And vice versa?

5. Time-based

a. What are your target dates for reaching discrete components of your goal? What do you plan to accomplish within:

◊ Today?
◊ A week?
◊ A month?
◊ Six months?
◊ A year?

Exercise 18-3: Setting Goals, Part 3—Future

This part of the exercise outlines the future—explicitly, how to be practical in order to achieve your goal. This step ties back to the previous step of establishing concrete steps for achieving your goal. Write down specific steps that underlie your strategy to obtain your goal. Here are points to consider:

1. *Foods.* Identify foods you want to eat and foods to avoid. While your choices may change over time, use what you know right now to do this exercise.

2. *Habits.* Identify habits about food and what to continue and what to stop. This course will offer more ideas but, again, use what you know right now.

3. *Schedule*. Create a schedule. Examples are: "Every day or every week, I will…"

4. *Kindness*. Devote yourself to kindness; this is not an all-or-nothing plan. Here are sample statements. "I will be kind to myself and know I am doing my best." "If I forget one day, I will take a deep breath and remind myself to try again." "I can adjust the list if needed."

5. *Flexibility*. Build flexibility into your plan such as "five out of seven days."

6. *Duration*. Set a time period such as "for duration of the course," "for two weeks," or "by the next doctor's visit."

7. *Awareness*. Acknowledge any improvements such as when you walk farther than the week before or your blood pressure is improved or sleep is more restful.

8. *Accountability*. Maintain accountability. Write into your plan that you will consult with your doctor or health practitioner (if necessary). Post the list in a noticeable place and track your progress.

I used specific tactics to accomplish my three goals (stated previously) that coincide with these steps. (My age at the time is noted parenthetically.)

Goal (early 20s). "I want to have more energy to get my work done."

Tactics. Stabilize my daily routine. Eat food on a regular basis. Eat grains, beans, and vegetables regularly. Stop my addiction to snack foods.

Goal (30s). "I want to be healthy to keep up with my boys."

Tactics. Make breakfast by a certain time. Include foods they will eat and that nourish me. Exercise with them such as ride bikes, hike in woods, or play baseball. Have story time every day. Plan the mid-afternoon snack consistently.

Goal (40s). "I want my intuition to flourish."

Tactics. Take time to meditate every day. Align my schedule with work, exercise, eating, and recreation. Get out with girlfriends frequently—at least 3 times a month.

Goal (of a friend of mine with cancer): "I want to reduce the severity of the disease and have less pain."

Tactics. Eat healthy foods every day. Chew each mouthful 100 to 200 times. Walk six out of seven days, if only to mailbox. Continue to monitor my health with my doctor.

You can be as extensive as you wish with these goals and tactics; either writing a long-term outline or a quick plan for your immediate needs. Either way, bear in mind that it takes about six weeks to establish a new habit or replace an old one. Use this exercise to help you plan SMART goals that fit with where you are right now and with what you want to change.

Summary

Planning for the future is a big deal. It requires optimism that you can achieve the things important to you. Pat yourself on the back for stating objectives, goals, and tactics, and for looking at where you've been and what you hope to accomplish next. This book is designed to help you meet your goals—goals based on what is important and achievable for you. Let food be your support. Let intuition be your guide.

Nutrition: The Foundation of Practice

Nutrition supports your health and vitality.
Your common sense about nutrition enables
you to take care of yourself.

In this unit, you learn that eating nutritious foods that you enjoy will provide satisfaction. These two—nutrition and satisfaction—stem from a commonsense approach to eating, which strengthens your intuitive awareness.

Keyword: Common Sense

The main objective of this unit is to appreciate the value of common sense. Nutrition is not rocket science, but it is built on ideas that make sense. When you apply common sense to nutrition, you notice how foods satisfy you—a knowledge that strengthens your intuitive ability about nutrition.

Food: Specific Foods to Eat

Tailor your food consumption to align with the concepts in this unit. Eat healthy food; the lessons suggest specific foods to eat.

Exercise: Plan Menus to Coincide with Lessons

This exercise prepares you for the lessons in this unit:

1. Use the *Life Template* from Lesson 7 to preview your work

responsibilities, family duties, recreational activities, and available time for meal preparation.

2. Use *Menu Template* from Lesson 7 to plan meals that include quality foods each day.

3. Include any food goals that you set in Lesson 18, as appropriate.

4. Lesson 20 covers carbohydrates. Include a piece of fruit for that day, specific to the exercise, and a complex carbohydrate from whole grain. These two items can be at separate meals.

5. Lesson 21 covers protein. Include beans or animal protein, specific to that day, in order to complete the exercise.

6. Lesson 22 covers fats. Include sautéed vegetables or a salad with drizzled salad dressing and nuts for a snack, again specific to the exercise.

7. Lesson 23 covers vitamins and minerals. Plan an assortment of colorful foods for that day.

Note: Theory without practice is all words. Practice without theory has no focus. You need both: theory (information) and practice (experience). Menu planning is a practical exercise built from ideas. Each unit from now on contains a menu planning exercise to practice the ideas. By the end of this course, you will have gained much experience; more importantly, you will possess profound knowledge about your desires, preferences, and intuition.

Resources: Appendix 4
◊ *Glycemic Index*
◊ *Protein Needs for Optimum Diet*
◊ *Summary of Vitamins and Minerals*
◊ *Weight Loss or Gain*

Getting Started: Lessons 19 to 24

Carbohydrate, Proteins, and Fats—you've probably heard these words a million times. We are overloaded with nutritional information; requirements, recommendations, and labels are everywhere. In this unit, you learn how to navigate through it all using a common-sense approach.

Lesson 19

Nutrition

Tap into what you already know and
activate your intuition.

Nutrition ensured the successful evolution of humankind and is the reason we have thrived for millennia. Basic intake of calories ensures sustenance; however, proper nutrition is required for the long-term health of the species. The earliest humans—scavengers, hunters, and gatherers—moved around to find a variety of food sources. They knew the importance of nutrients. An essential turning point for humans was the cultivation of food to ensure sufficient and consistent nutrition.

Seeking proper nutrition to build a strong body is similar to obtaining proper materials to build a house. The builder uses quality materials such as stone, wood, and metal to provide a stable foundation and strong internal supports. Likewise, we seek quality foods to build strong bodies.

The exercise today recognizes the place nutrition has in your life. You write an *Ideal Menu Plan* using what you already know about nutrition. This exercise reinforces the idea that your intuition is working for you.

Exercise 19: Ideal Menu Plan

What do you love to eat? Not for taste, not for holidays, but for satisfaction. Think of the foods that nourish you so thoroughly that you say, "That was a perfect day of meals." For today, write down those menus. Elaborate on your ideal day of meals. You won't have to prepare it, but make the list complete, as we will refer to this plan for the rest of this unit. For this exercise:

1. Use a large sheet of paper or several sheets. Label four rows: Breakfast, Lunch, Dinner, and Snacks. Leave enough space between rows to accommodate additional notes for each meal.

2. List for each meal the foods that you most enjoy for that meal. In addition to flavors, think of colors, variety, and what you like to eat in combination. Make your list of foods as healthy and nutritious as possible.

3. Write one item, dish, or recipe per line. If it has multiple ingredients, keep a blank line after for notes.

4. Complete your list of ideal meals, including side dishes, toppings, sauces, garnishes, desserts, and other items that you love and that round out the meal.

5. Quantity doesn't matter, but note which meal is the largest meal of your day.

Summary

Your *Ideal Menu Plan* includes carbohydrates, proteins, fats, vitamins, and minerals because all foods have these to one degree or another. The lessons that come next elaborate on the nutritional details. Realize that you already know something about which foods provide which nutrients. This awareness reinforces your intuitive understanding of the link between nutrition and satisfaction.

Lesson 20

Carbohydrates

Carbohydrates are the fuel of humanity.

Carbohydrates are macronutrients; that is, nutrients that humans need in large amounts. Proteins and fats are the other macronutrients. Carbohydrates provide energy—the "fuel" that keeps a person going. Just as your car needs the right fuel, you need the right carbohydrates to feel good and have energy to do what you want.

Energy comes from glucose—the basic unit of carbohydrates. Plants make glucose by photosynthesis, turning light energy into food energy. Plants store glucose in roots, seeds, and fruits as sugars and starches that keep your body going. Glucose feeds the brain, activates muscles, and operates the basic bodily processes of digestion, respiration, circulation, and elimination. Although glucose is a form of sugar, it is very different from white refined sugar.

Carbon, hydrogen, and oxygen form a ring of glucose that bands together in chains with other rings of glucose to form carbohydrates. Short chains make simple carbohydrates; long chains make complex carbohydrates. Some of the short chains are fructose, found in fruits; lactose, found in milk; maltose, found in sprouted grains and beer; and sucrose, found in cane sugar and beet sugar. Long chains are found in cereal grains, beans, and starchy vegetables such as potatoes and sweet potatoes.

Humans benefit most from both simple and complex carbohydrates when they come from a healthy source that contains fiber, a specific type of carbohydrate that is hard to digest. Fiber is present in the cellular walls of plants, and it forms the bran of cereal grains, the skins of vegetables, and the roughage of fresh fruits. Fiber has no calories but is beneficial because it provides bulk for the stool, slows digestion (in a good way), and reduces the speed with which glucose enters the bloodstream. When fiber is present, a person gains energy in a steady way—the glucose enters the bloodstream in a constant drip, so to speak. When carbohydrates are stripped of fiber (for example, white sugar, processed foods, sweetened drinks), glucose enters the bloodstream in a rush.

Glucose enters the bloodstream in various ways, depending on the carbohydrate. White refined sugar, the simplest form of a simple carbohydrate, releases glucose in the mouth the instant it encounters saliva, in which the enzyme ptyalin acts on carbohydrates to release glucose. Fruit, a simple carbohydrate containing some fiber, releases glucose in both the mouth and in the digestive tract. Whole grains, complex carbohydrates containing fiber, releases glucose both in the mouth and in the digestive tract. When you chew carbohydrates, your body reacts differently depending on whether or not the food is refined and which foods are eaten at the same time. For example, fruit baked in a pie provides glucose more slowly than fruit juice. The Glycemic Index (*Appendix 4*) shows the speeds at which carbohydrates are converted to glucose in the body.

The following exercises elaborate on carbohydrates and how to use intuition to experience them.

Exercise 20-1: Identify Carbohydrates on the Menu Plan

Using the *Ideal Menu Plan* you created in Lesson 19, mark each item as directed below. You can mark items more than once. Do your best to identify all carbohydrates, especially in recipes that have multiple ingredients.

1. Mark the following items with "CC" for complex carbohydrates.
   ◊ Whole grains such as brown rice, millet, buckwheat, whole oats, quinoa, teff, and amaranth.
   ◊ Grain products such as whole wheat or other bread, corn tortillas, rolled oats or oatmeal, crackers, and whole-grain flatbreads, muffins, or pasta. Also include granola and

boxed cereals (if they contain whole grains), and snacks
such as popcorn or cookies (if they contain whole-grain
flour).
◊ Beans such as pintos, black beans, green split peas, and
others.
◊ Nuts, seeds, and nut or seed butters.
◊ All vegetables such as starchy tubers (sweet potatoes or
potatoes), cabbage family (broccoli and cabbage), and
roots (carrots and onions).

2. Mark the following items with one "C" for simple carbohydrate.
◊ Fresh whole fruits.
◊ Refined grains and grain products such as white rice, cous-
cous, and white pasta.
◊ Foods that contain refined white flour.
◊ Boxed cereals (if they do not contain whole grains).
◊ Sweeteners such as maple syrup, honey, barley malt, and
rice syrup. Do not mark refined sugar.
◊ Concentrated fruits such as jams, dried fruits, and fruit
leathers.
◊ Fruit juices, beer, or wine.

3. Mark the following foods with an "XC" for the simplest carbohydrates.
◊ Any items that contain refined white or brown sugar,
including candies, pies, cakes, and store-bought pre-pack-
aged foods.
◊ Any items that contain high-fructose corn syrup or artificial sweeteners such as aspartame or xylitol.

Exercise 20-2: Consume Simple Carbohydrate
Take a bite of fresh fruit such as an apple, a pear, or a peach for
a snack. Eat that bite as you normally eat fruit. Then, take a second
bite; as you chew it, hold it in your mouth longer than the first bite.
Compare the second bite with the first and observe your reaction. Do

you notice a difference? What happens to your saliva? How is the taste? How does your body react? Immediately? Over the next hour?

Exercise 20-3: Consume Complex Carbohydrate.

Take a bite of a whole grain such as brown rice at a meal. Eat that bite as you normally would. Then, take a second bite; as you chew it, hold it in your mouth longer than the first bite. Compare the second bite with the first. Observe your reaction. Do you notice a difference? What happens to your saliva? How is the taste? How does your body react? Immediately? Over the next hour?

Exercise 20-4: Note Energy Level

Reflect for a moment on your energy. Do you have steady energy over the day? Do you have ups and downs? If you started eating more complex carbohydrates since beginning this course, have you noticed any difference?

Summary

Complex carbohydrates provide steady and consistent energy for your body. Your intuition helps you sense them, both in flavor and in your bodily reaction. Quality carbohydrates strengthen your health and your intuition, and intuition helps you choose the appropriate carbohydrates, a wonderful self-sustaining cycle.

Lesson 21

Proteins

Protein provides mass for the body.

Protein is a macronutrient needed for growth, especially during childhood and adolescence. It builds muscles, helps repair injuries, and makes up most of body weight that is not water. Protein is found in internal cells, tissues, lymph, and some hormones.

Proteins are similar to carbohydrates in that both have carbon, oxygen, and hydrogen. Proteins also have nitrogen. These four elements come together in specific forms to create amino acids, the building blocks of protein. The body can reassemble amino acids into carbon, oxygen, and hydrogen for glucose and energy need. However, when this occurs, the unused nitrogen must be metabolized by the liver and kidneys, which creates stress on these organs. Thus, many doctors and nutritionists feel it is better to rely on carbohydrate for everyday energy rather than protein.

There are 20 amino acids; 10 are essential and must be provided by food. When a person obtains these 10, the body can assemble the others. One special class of proteins is enzymes, chains of amino acids that aid in converting sugars to glucose, assimilating vitamin B_{12}, or utilizing insulin.

Protein is found in all sources of unprocessed foods. Fish, meat, and beans have many amino acids, but plants such as mushrooms and lettuce contain some amino acids too. Animal foods contain a high proportion of protein, as do beans and legumes. Seeds, nuts, and grains have smaller proportions; their amino acid profiles complement beans and legumes. Together they comprise amino acid profiles comparable to those found in eggs or meats. *Diet for a Small Planet*, authored in the early 1970s by Frances Moore Lappé, was one of the first books to chart and popularize this data. She encouraged people to eat beans and grains at the same meal for optimum health.

Through the years, nutritionists have supported or opposed this research. Some agree but say that vegetarians need to be vigilant in eating grains and beans simultaneously; others disagree and say it is not that difficult, nor is it necessary, to obtain protein exclusively from plant sources. The need for protein varies greatly from individual to individual and from time to time—some people need higher quantities to function well; other people function best on lower amounts. A person's age, general health, and activity level impact which protein sources are best for that individual. Some disorders require that a person monitor her/his protein intake, and other conditions may necessitate consuming more protein. Finally, there are ethical and spiritual considerations as to which protein sources to consume. For all of these reasons, people develop preferences for different sources of protein.

Optimum protein consumption depends on three things: eating the quantity that is adequate for you, as an individual; obtaining the protein from reasonable sources; and preparing the protein in ways that are practical and pleasurable. The exercise today elaborates on these details. For more information, see *Appendix 4.*

Exercise 21-1: Identify Protein on Menu Plan

On the *Ideal Menu Plan* that you created in Exercise 19, identify the major sources of protein.

1. Mark the following foods with a "PP" for preferred sources of protein.
   ◊ Beans such as pinto beans, black beans, garbanzo beans, lentils, and nigari tofu (contains magnesium chloride).
   ◊ Products containing beans such as soy sauce or miso only if they are consumed in a sizable portion, such as two tablespoons or more.
   ◊ Nuts, seeds, or their butters, if consumed in a sizable portion such as two tablespoons.
   ◊ Do not label grains, vegetables, or starchy roots. While these foods contain protein, it is considered a minor source for this exercise.

2. Identify the following sources of protein and mark with "P" for sources that are very good, but not ones to consume every day—in my opinion.
   ◊ Animal foods such as organic beef, chicken, pork, turkey, and wild-caught fish either as a main course or as a component of another dish. Do not mark foods that are not

labeled organic.
◊ Eggs if consumed in a sufficient portion. For example, scrambled eggs constitute a major source of protein; one egg used in a batch of 24 muffins does not.
◊ Packaged tofu that includes additional ingredients beyond soybeans, water, and nigari. (Nigari is often labeled as magnesium chloride.)
◊ Soy foods that are not labeled as organic. Almost all non-organic soybeans are genetically modified. Manufacturers who use organic soybeans label the package; sometimes they note *GMO-free*. Assume the soy is genetically modified if the product is not labeled organic.

3. Identify the following sources of protein and mark with "XP" for sources best to avoid.
◊ Animal foods that are not organic.
◊ Packaged animal foods such as lunch meats, hot dogs, or beef jerky that contain preservatives and excess sodium.
◊ Meat from fast-food stores or meat that is deep fried.

Because dairy foods contain more grams of fat than grams of protein, they constitute a minor source of protein and are not included in this exercise.

Exercise 21-2: Consume Protein

Consume a quality protein (PP or P) dish today. Choose either a plant- or animal-based source. One serving is one-half cup of cooked beans, two eggs, or four ounces of meat, about the size of a deck of cards. Balance the meal with other foods.

Chew one bite of the protein dish thoroughly. Notice your reaction to flavor. When I do this exercise, beans taste sweet with more chewing. Meat is the opposite—it tastes less delicious with longer chewing. What is your experience?

Exercise 21-3: Note Core Energy

Consider how much core energy, or stamina, you have. Carbohydrates are fuel to use throughout the day; protein is like the battery that gets you started. Do you have abundant energy? Or are you tired all the time or frequently during the day?

If you feel depleted in the core of your body, you probably need more protein. The way to tell if you are depleted rather than tired is to pay attention to your energy level when you wake in the morning. If you are depleted, you drag all day; if you are tired, you pick up when you eat. Also, pay attention to how you recover from illness. If you are depleted, it takes longer to bounce back.

Summary

Protein is in your muscles. You can notice protein as a source of energy by the stamina it provides. Tap into your intuition to reflect honestly on your protein needs. Use your intuition to determine your preferred protein sources. For additional information about protein for an optimum diet, see *Appendix 4*.

Lesson 22

Fats

Fats. Despite negative connotations, this substance is vital for your body's growth. Fats are to be celebrated, not denigrated.

Fats are one of the macronutrients needed for life. Like carbohydrates and proteins, they are a source of energy. Carbohydrates provide everyday energy; proteins, core energy; and fats, reserve energy.

Humans (and animals) depend on fats as a storehouse for energy, for growth, and for survival through lean times. Fats are concentrated nutrition, more dense than protein. The body uses fats for metabolism, as building blocks for cell membranes and hormones, and for warmth and insulation of the internal organs. Fats make up a large portion of the brain, they lubricate the cells, and they help retain moisture in the skin. Fats are extremely important for growth, especially in babies and children who need a larger quantity than adults. Fats also give flavor to food and satisfaction in meals by slowing down nutrient absorption. As a result, we feel full longer if we eat an appropriate amount of fat.

However, there are dangers relative to the quantity and quality of fats consumed. The national obesity problem in the U.S. stems in large measure from excess consumption of poor-quality fats combined with excess simple carbohydrates and sugars, particularly in soft drinks. Although, adults need fats in their diets, it is critical to good health to choose the right fats, avoid the wrong ones, and be vigilant about limiting how much is consumed.

There are different kinds of fats. Depending on their chemical composition, they are classified as saturated, monounsaturated, or polyunsaturated. An easy way to determine which type you have is by whether the fat is solid or liquid at room temperature and when chilled. For example, butter and other animal fats are solid at room temperature; thus, they are saturated fats. Vegetable oils such as sesame or flax remain liquid when chilled; thus, they are polyunsaturated. Olive oil is liquid at room temperature and solid when chilled; thus, it is a monounsaturated fat.

Fats are further classified by their structure and length. Fats are made of fatty acids, chains of carbon atoms with hydrogen atoms filling the bonds. All available carbon bonds of saturated fatty acids are occupied by hydrogen atoms. They form straight, short chains that are stable and not easily broken apart during heating.

Monounsaturated fatty acids have chains with some kinks in them—places where two carbon atoms bond with each other and two hydrogen atoms are missing. The kink in the chain makes these fats more fluid, yet still relatively stable. These chains don't break apart or denature (become rancid) very easily. Chains of monounsaturated fatty acids are medium to long in length.

Polyunsaturated fatty acids have more than one kink in the chain, and they form long to very long chains of atoms. These chains are unstable and break apart easily. This becomes important when oils are extracted in production and when used in cooking and baking. Polyunsaturated oils are more perishable than saturated or monounsaturated oils.

Vegetal sources of fats are mainly in the seeds of plants, whether the actual seed, a nut from a tree, or the germ of a bean or grain. This seed contains a storehouse of nutrients for a new plant to grow. When a seed sprouts, the emerging sprout uses the fat as a source of energy. This fat supplies enough nutrients for the sprout to become large enough to manufacture its own energy through its leaves and roots. Animal sources of fats come from dairy foods and meats.

It is important to include fats in your diet, to use quality sources, and to avoid overheating when cooking so they won't denature. Today's exercise elaborates on fats to help you identify and experience them in your foods.

Exercise 22-1: Identify Fats on Menu Plan

On your *Ideal Menu Plan*, identify the major sources of fat. Any quantity used counts.

1. Identify the following fat sources and mark with an "FF" for healthy sources of fat, ones that are okay to eat every day.
   ◊ Nuts such as walnuts and almonds or nut butters such as almond butter and peanut butter.
   ◊ Seeds such as sesame seeds, sunflower seeds, and pumpkin seeds or seed butters such as tahini.
   ◊ Any foods or dishes that contain organic unrefined oils, such as extra virgin olive oil used in salad dressings or sesame oil used in cooking.
   ◊ Organic unrefined oils used as supplements such as flax or fish oil.

2. Identify the following fat sources and mark with an "F" for healthy sources of fats, but not ones to have every day.
   ◊ Organic butter, ghee, and dairy foods, including organic whole milk.
   ◊ Organic meats, poultry, eggs, and fish.
   ◊ Organic unrefined extra virgin coconut oil used in any dish.
   ◊ Homemade fried foods using quality oils.
   ◊ Homemade desserts using quality oils.

3. Identify the following fat sources and mark with an "XF" for less than ideal sources of fat that should be avoided.
   ◊ Commercially raised animal foods and dairy foods, especially ice cream.
   ◊ Any foods or dishes that contain refined canola oil, corn oil, cottonseed oil, peanut oil, safflower oil, soy oil, or other oil that doesn't state it is organic and unrefined.
   ◊ Packaged foods that contain any of the oils listed above, such as chips, crackers, cookies, granola, etc. *Note*: Even health food stores carry products that contain refined oils.
   ◊ Food eaten in restaurants. Very few restaurants use quality fats in production due to the high cost. Unless you are certain of the integrity of the kitchen, assume the oil is cheap and not very healthy.

Although grains and beans contain fat, it is in much smaller amounts than carbohydrates and protein and only a minor source. Therefore, for this exercise, they are not included.

Exercise 22-2: Consume Plant-Based Fat

Fats provide richness and taste appeal. Consume quality fats today according to the following suggestions:

1. Use olive oil in salad dressing at one meal today, or sauté vegetables in a small amount of sesame oil. Chew well when eating,

noting the flavor of the dish. Salads taste better when accompanied by dressing; vegetables are delicious when lightly sautéed. Pay particular attention to the length of time that passes before you get hungry again. Fats slow digestion so you may be surprised at how long it is before you want another meal.

2. Eat nuts such as almonds, pecans, and walnuts or sunflower seeds for a snack today. Chew very well to grind them up and mix with your saliva. Notice the difference in the flavor. Nuts and seeds contain fats and carbohydrates, and the flavor increases with chewing. Also, note if you eat less when you chew more. Pay attention to your level of satisfaction and how much time passes before you are hungry again.

Exercise 22-3: Note Energetic Storehouse

Your fat reserves in your body are a storehouse of energy for when you need a substantial boost, such as during cold winters, famines, and pregnancy for women. You can gauge the volume of this energy storehouse by your reaction to fasting. A person without fat reserves often feels worse when fasting. A person with adequate reserves feels energized. Recall your reaction to your limited fast in Lesson 16. Did you feel better afterwards? Or did you feel tired the next day?

Summary

Fats are a storehouse of energy, necessary for survival, growth, and health. They provide richness to meals and a bounty of nutrition for times when you need a boost. Your intuition helps you determine your need for fats, and your body's reaction provides feedback to your intuition. Cultivate your intuition about fats to decide what to use and how often. For more details, refer to *Appendix 3: Intuition about Oils*.

Lesson 23

Vitamins and Minerals

Be mindful of the little things. With this mindfulness comes the realization that there are no little things—nothing is insignificant.

Vitamins and minerals are micronutrients required by the body. Similar to the macronutrients (carbohydrates, proteins, and fats), vitamins and minerals are also concentrations of energy and nutrients, providing small but vital amounts. You can think of them like booster shots, which supply medicine in a small, concentrated dose. Vitamins and minerals do a lot of internal work such as helping with metabolism, growth, respiration, and digestion. They are little powerhouses that take care of the minutiae of the body, helping the body run smoothly like a well-oiled machine.

Different foods provide various vitamins and minerals. Some vitamins and minerals are found in vegetal foods, others in animal foods, and others in both vegetal and animal foods.

Vitamins are classified as either water soluble or fat soluble. Water-soluble vitamins (C and B complex) help regulate enzyme reactions in processing carbohydrates, proteins, and fats. They are eliminated through normal excretion (respiration and elimination). The fat-soluble vitamins (A, D, E, and K) are accumulated in the fatty tissues and stored for later use. Because they are retained in the body, excess intake of vitamin A and vitamin D, especially if synthetic, can be toxic.

Minerals support numerous bodily functions—from comprising the structure of bones and tissues to helping balance acidity and alkalinity in bodily fluids. There are 28 naturally occurring essential minerals. Unless your diet is severely restricted, minerals are easily available in whole foods. Your body uses seven of them (calcium, chlorine, magnesium, phosphorous, potassium, sodium, and sulfur) in greater amounts than the remainder, which fall into the category of trace minerals.

Whole natural foods naturally provide a wealth of nutrients. It is easy to obtain adequate vitamins and minerals if your diet includes a variety of foods. The summary of the most used vitamins and minerals, including primary sources and functions, is in *Appendix 4*.

Exercise 23-1: Identify Vitamins and Minerals on Your Menu Plan

Mark the following sources of vitamins and minerals on your *Ideal Menu Plan* (created in Exercise 19). Make a mark any time they appear, even if in a very small amount (such as one egg in a batch of 24 muffins of which you eat one). By now, your *Ideal Menu Plan* is probably accumulating a lot of marks—an indication of a diverse diet. Mark the food items using the following symbols:

◊ "VA" for vitamin A in eggs, butter, or fish oils.
◊ "VA" also for beta carotene in carrots, winter squash, sweet potatoes, apricots, and greens such as spinach and beet greens.
◊ "VB" for vitamin B complex (thiamine, riboflavin, and niacin usually accompany each other) in whole grains, legumes, nuts, and seeds.
◊ "VB12" for vitamin B_{12} in animal foods, dairy products, eggs, or supplements.
◊ "VC" for vitamin C in citrus and other fruits, broccoli and green leafy vegetables eaten raw or lightly cooked.
◊ "VD" for vitamin D in fish oils, organic butter, eggs, fortified milk and other dairy products and if you spend 15 minutes or more in sunlight daily.
◊ "VE" for vitamin E in nuts, seeds, whole grains, and whole-grain breads.
◊ "CA" for calcium in dairy products, green leafy vegetables, seaweed, and sesame seeds.

◊ "F" for folic acid in leafy greens.
◊ "FE" for iron in red meat, prunes, figs, raisins, and sea-
   weeds.
◊ "I" for iodine in seafood, seaweed, and sea salt.
◊ "MLT" for nutritional supplements. If you take isolated
   ones, label accordingly.

Although there are more minerals and phytochemicals, this exercise is meant to identify major groups of micronutrients rather than listing all of them.

Exercise 23-2: Consume Ample Fruits and Vegetables

Aim to eat nine servings of fruits and vegetables per day, a serving being the equivalent of ½ cup cooked broccoli, one cup of salad, or ½ large apple. Include at least five servings of vegetables. Use a variety of types and colors, according to the following color spectrum:

◊ *Red*. Beets, red bell pepper, tomatoes, radish, strawberry,
   cherry, watermelon.
◊ *Orange*. Carrot, winter squash, rutabaga, mango, oranges.
◊ *Yellow*. Yellow squash, spaghetti squash, parsnips, corn on
   the cob, lemon.
◊ *White*. Onion, garlic, bok choy (white part), mushrooms,
   cauliflower, cucumber, banana.
◊ *Green*. Kale, collards, mustard greens, lettuce, broccoli,
   bok choy (green part), parsley, celery, cucumber, green
   bell pepper, peas, watercress, zucchini.
◊ *Blue*. Blueberries.
◊ *Purple*. Eggplant, plums, grapes.
◊ *Black/brown*. Mushrooms, seaweeds such as arame, dulse,
   hijiki (hiziki), kombu, nori, spirulina, wakame.

This list of vegetables and fruits is not exhaustive—feel free to include other fruits and vegetables as desired.

Here is one example of how to include 9 servings of vegetables and fruits in one day of meals. (Serving number is denoted in parentheses.)

◊ *Breakfast*. Berries (1), toast, whole-grain cooked cereal.
◊ *Lunch*. Sandwich that includes lettuce, tomato, and sprouts (1), whole apple (2).
◊ *Snack*. Carrot and cucumber sticks (1), raisins (1), nuts, rice cakes.
◊ *Dinner*. Soup with vegetables (1), rice, stir-fried vegetables (2)

Exercise 23-3: Note Energetic Boost

Pay attention to how you feel once you have started eating more fruits and vegetables on a regular basis. If you didn't previously eat many vegetables regularly, you may notice anything from feeling lighter to feeling more exuberant. If you do eat many vegetables on a regular basis, focus on the variety of colors and how appealing they are to you.

Summary

Vitamins and minerals are abundant in a well-balanced, whole foods diet. Vitamins and minerals enhance your health, which in turn heightens your intuition. Let your intuition flourish by eating a diet high in nutrients; in turn, your intuition will help you select nutritious foods.

Lesson 24

REVIEW: **Nutrition: The Foundation of Practice**

The optimum diet is one that works today and every day.

This is a time to review and create your optimum diet. In this unit, you learned to recognize that you want satisfaction from your food and that nutritious foods provide maximum satisfaction. With this information, you can design a diet that works for you—an optimum diet that is nutritionally balanced and one that meets your physical need for energy and your emotional need for satisfaction.

The lessons in this unit offer a perspective on nutrition as the source of energy—both for the physical body and for emotional satisfaction. Energy is the link between nutrition and satisfaction.

Here are summaries of the five lessons:

Lesson 19: Nutrition. You wrote an *Ideal Menu Plan* of nutritious foods you love to eat.

Lesson 20: Carbohydrates. Carbohydrates are the fuel for your everyday energy.

Lesson 21: Proteins. Proteins provide muscle mass for your core energy.

Lesson 22: Fats. Fats store reserve energy for times when you have extra needs (illness, extreme weather, pregnancy).

Lesson 23: Vitamins and Minerals. Vitamins and minerals add sparks of energy to fuel your exuberance.

Following are the foods suggested to supply these nutrients:

Carbohydrates
◊ Organic whole grains and beans (complex carbohydrates).
◊ Organic vegetables (complex carbohydrates).
◊ Organic fruits (simple carbohydrates).
◊ All whole foods contain fiber.

Protein
◊ Whole or split, organic beans and dried peas.
◊ Organic nuts, seeds, and organic nut and seed butters (in reasonable portions).
◊ Grains and beans (consumed at same meal).
◊ Organic fish and animal foods (in reasonable portions, if consumed at all).

Fats
◊ Organic nuts, seeds, and organic nut and seed butters (in reasonable portions).
◊ Organic unrefined oils.
◊ Organic unsalted butter and/or organic dairy foods (if consumed at all).

Vitamins and Minerals
◊ Whole foods for fiber (whether grain bran and germ, bean, vegetable, or fruit).
◊ Organic foods for higher quantities of vitamins and minerals.
◊ Colorful fruits and vegetables for abundance of nutrients.
◊ Sea vegetables and sea salt for minerals.
◊ Supplements as needed.

Keep these foods in mind as you design your optimal diet.

Exercise 24-1: Optimal Diet
The optimal diet is one that works—today, tomorrow, in the fu-

ture. It works because it addresses the following needs that everyone has:

Practical. An optimal diet works throughout your life. When you plan menus that fit with your schedule, responsibilities, and activities, you have a diet that is realistic. Consider the menu plan you created in this unit that took into account your work, hobbies, activities, and family responsibilities.

Physical. An optimal diet works for your health. When you include appropriate nutrition in proper quantities, you have a diet that gives you energy. Consider how you proceeded through the *Ideal Menu Plan* to incorporate nutrition.

Emotional. An optimal diet works for your comfort. When you eat foods you enjoy, you are satisfied and are motivated to maintain this practice. Consider how you brainstormed for the *Ideal Menu Plan* to choose foods you love.

Mental. An optimal diet works for your mind. When you learn about food, cooking, menu planning, nutrition, and other details, you grow. Consider what you learned in this unit.

Spiritual. An optimal diet works for your integration. Many things you do provide benefits on many levels. Remember: when you plan menus, you are being proactive in meeting your practical, physical, emotional, and mental needs. And, when you sit down to slowly and thoughtfully chew your food, you focus on being in the moment, thereby helping your body, emotions, and mind.

Exercise 24-2: Optimal Diet—Review *Ideal Menu Plan*

For this exercise, review your *Ideal Menu Plan* and evaluate how well you did. Look at your plan and all the notations you made. Optimally, you included complex carbohydrates, protein, fats, vitamins, and minerals from fruits, vegetables, seeds, beans, and grains. Is there any nutrient that was overemphasized or is glaringly missing?

Exercise 24-3: Optimal diet—Energy level

How much energy do you have? How much do you need? Here is a summary from the lessons:

Carbohydrates provide everyday energy. If you are consuming the right quantity, you have consistent energy throughout the day and can do everything you want to do without drastic swings in blood sugar. If you have mood swings or shifts in energy, you probably need to eat more complex carbohydrates regularly throughout the day.

Proteins provide core energy. If you are consuming the proper amount, whether animal or vegetal, you have stamina. If you are fatigued beyond what would be considered normal for someone your age, you may need more protein.

Fats provide reserve energy and satisfaction. Fats stick with you. If you are eating the correct amount, you will be able to do a short-term fast without exhaustion. If you are hungry too soon after a meal, you need more fats. If you feel sluggish, you may need less fat in your diet.

Vitamins and minerals come from all foods. Fresh vegetables and fruits provide exuberance, spirit, and liveliness. If you are consuming the right quantity, you feel alert and refreshed. If you need more perkiness, eat more fruits and vegetables.

Here are general guidelines for certain situations:

◊ *Illness.* If you have any disease, your food and water must be as healthy and as free from toxins as possible. Eat complex carbohydrates and not too many simple carbohydrates from fruit or juices. Eat whole foods so you have fiber. Avoid refined carbohydrates, especially white flour, white sugar, artificial sweeteners, and candy. Choose quality protein from plant-based sources. Limit animal protein including dairy foods and, if consumed, choose organic products. Obtain fats through nuts, seeds, and small amounts of unrefined oils. Avoid all fried foods. Use supplements if your doctor recommends them.

◊ *Health*. Consume high quality/organic carbohydrates, proteins, and unrefined fats in sufficient proportions. Eat a wide variety of foods to ensure plenty of vitamins and minerals. Drink an adequate amount of good-quality water.

◊ *Physical work*. Eat more protein to increase stamina.

◊ *Mental work*. Eat sufficient complex carbohydrates; avoid excess simple carbohydrates.

◊ *Deep sleep*. Eat carbohydrates, proteins, and fats throughout the day; eat less protein and fats at the last meal of the day.

◊ *Athletic performance*. Eat an equal ratio of protein to carbohydrate. If you are training, whole grains and beans without excess simple carbohydrates can build up muscle tone and endurance.

◊ *Sexual satisfaction*. Consume all nutrients in the proper proportion. Avoid too much fat. Some people need more protein for stamina. Others need fruits and vegetables to be more open.

◊ *Constipation*. Eat fiber, particularly by consuming whole fruits and vegetables.

◊ *Loose stools*. Eat whole grains and beans.

◊ *Hungry after eating*. Eat more fat and complex carbohydrates.

◊ *Heavy feeling after eating*. Eat more vegetables and less fat.

◊ *Pregnant women. Children. Teenagers*. Eat more protein, fats, and vitamins and minerals than carbohydrates.

◊ *Weight loss or weight gain*. See *Appendix 4* for suggestions.

Exercise 24-4: Optimal Diet — How to Design Yours

Now that you have read what, theoretically, constitutes an optimal diet and evaluated your menu plan and energy level, you are ready for the comprehensive four-step plan for implementation.

1. *Daily nutrition*. Get basic nutrition every day from these sources.
 ◊ Carbohydrates from whole grains and organic vegetables and fruits.
 ◊ Protein from whole beans and small amounts of organic animal foods (if desired).
 ◊ Fats from nuts, seeds, unrefined vegetable oils, and small amounts of organic animal foods (if desired).
 ◊ Vitamins and minerals from a large variety of organic foods.

2. *Proportions*. Incorporate all nutrients in a reasonable proportion and avoid trendy diets (low-fat, high protein, or low simple-carbohydrate).
 ◊ *This is very important*: While you may need to consume low fat or high protein for awhile, avoid singling out one macronutrient at the expense of the others—especially for an extended period of time.
 ◊ If one category is consistently missing, such as never eating fat, it creates a hole in your nutritive needs, and your body will begin to suffer. Cravings begin, satisfaction lessens, health diminishes, and, over time, deficiencies arise.
 ◊ Regarding proportions, here is a reference point that I use for my largest meal of the day: ½ cup cooked brown rice; ½ cup cooked beans; 1 cup vegetables, both cooked and raw; and 2 tablespoons of nuts or 1 tablespoon of oil.
  – Sometimes, I serve less quantity, other times more.
  – At some meals, I want a higher proportion of rice to beans, or beans to rice, or vegetables to rice/beans, etc.
  – Proportions are very easy to alter as you are serving.

3. *Energy requirements*. Let your energy dictate how to adjust the proportions.

◊ When you need more day-to-day energy, eat more complex carbohydrates.

◊ If your energy is depleted, eat protein.

◊ To ensure fullness after meals, eat an appropriate quantity of high-quality fats.

◊ If you're not sure what to eat, ask yourself, "Do I need more of this, of that?" Listen to your intuition for the answer and rely on it to tailor your diet.

4. *Adjustments*. Vary your diet by including different foods.

◊ Try new recipes.

◊ Rotate foods on a weekly basis, monthly basis, and seasonal basis.

◊ Avoid getting stuck in a rut as to what you eat and how much you eat.

◊ Continue learning, adapting details, and trusting your intuition; it provides feedback about what works.

◊ Join a dinner group or recipe club, start a potluck, or find another social avenue to ensure diversity in your diet.

Summary

An optimal diet is an overview of how best to feed yourself. It works for your lifestyle, meets your nutritional needs, and satisfies your body, mind, and spirit. Nutrition is the foundation for physical health and vitality, which are integral to your emotional, mental, and spiritual health and vitality. Remember the importance of nutrition in providing the satisfaction you desire. Let intuition be your guiding light in helping you achieve both vitality and satisfaction.

PRINCIPLES: THE FRAMEWORK OF DIET

Your diet is the framework of your practice.
Base your diet on principles.

In this unit, you learn specific diet organization concepts that go beyond simple nutrition. In the process, you learn how these concepts apply to areas in your life beyond food.

Keyword: Stability

The main goal of this unit is to recognize the importance of stability in helping your mind and body thrive. Principles stabilize your mind by providing rational reasons for including or excluding foods. Principles stabilize your body by establishing habits that, over time, further stabilize your mind. Having stability of both your body and your mind will encourage your intuition to flourish—if you conscientiously apply principles.

Food: Old and New

During this unit, consume food according to the ideas presented previously. Coordinate what you have already learned with the new ideas presented in the following lessons.

Exercise: Plan Menus to Coincide with Lessons

This exercise prepares you for the lessons in this unit:

1. Use the *Life Template* from Lesson 7 to preview your work responsibilities, family duties, recreational activities, and

available time for meal preparation.

2. Use *Menu Template* from Lesson 7 to plan meals that include quality foods each day.

3. For Lesson 25 or Lesson 26, cook brown rice, prepared without soaking.

4. For Lesson 27, cook brown rice, prepared with soaking.

5. For Lesson 28, include a natural pickle to accompany the grain—see the lesson if needed.

6. For Lesson 29, plan a menu with good food combinations. Refer to *Cultural Menus* in *Appendix 5*.

7. For Lesson 30, plan a flavorful menu.

Resources: Appendix 5
◊ *Nutrition Menus*
◊ *Menus with Timings*
◊ *Celebration Menus*
◊ *Cultural Menus*
◊ *Intuition about Sprouts*
◊ *Intuition about Fermented Foods.*

Note: There are a number of menus in the appendices that model the ideas in this book. I encourage you to use them to create your own meals. As you prepare and consume your meals, continue to evaluate your experiences, note your reactions, and validate your intuitive awareness.

Getting Started: Lessons 25 to 30
Everyone knows what it is to be stable, to walk on two feet, or have balance between work and play. In the following lessons, you learn about creating stability in your diet by using principles that help establish order and create focus—in both your meals and your life.

Lesson 25

Continuation

*Continuation is the thread that links
experiences together.*

Everyone understands continuation. It is an organic principle, similar to breathing, that is reflected in the concept of life being a journey, continuing from day to day. Continuation can also be applied to food and your relationship to food.

Exercise 25-1: Grain and Continuation

A plant with a specific life cycle, grains are literally an example of continuity. They are the seeds that sprout, send down roots, grow leaves and stalks, and shoot up to grow in the sunshine, where they absorb light and manufacture food through photosynthesis. As the plant grows, it flowers, pollinates, and produces another seed. When the seed falls onto the ground or is planted, the cycle repeats.

Grains, the seeds of plants, begin and end the cycle; they are the first and last product in the life of the plant. When we eat grains, we become part of this continuous cycle. Being nourished by a food that is both the beginning and the end creates a pattern in our own energetic cycle that replicates this continuation.

For this exercise, eat a whole grain at one of your meals today and consider the continuity that you have ingested. This is a powerful concept!

Exercise 25-2: Dietary Continuation

The foods/diets you have eaten over the years have formed your current relationship with food. For this exercise, review any specific diet(s) you followed in the past and answer the following questions about each one:

1. What was the diet?

2. How did it help you at the time?

3. Why did you start eating this way?

4. Were you able to maintain the diet?

5. What is a long-term benefit or lesson you received from this diet?

6. If you haven't used any specific diets, what has been your general approach to food?

7. How has this approach helped you?

Many people adopt or change diets for various reasons:
◊ Health, such as a desire to lower cholesterol
◊ Vegetarian, to avoid eating meat
◊ Fast food, for convenience
◊ An all-or-nothing attitude; stopping a diet because it was hard to do perfectly

These ways of thinking are reactive, limiting, and, if you consider it further, inaccurate.

Each time you change your diet, it is due to an intuitive need to help yourself. Considered this way, you realize that your approach to food is an evolution of your dietary consciousness because each prior experience has contributed to your pool of knowledge. This is the basis of your intuitive awareness.

Finish this exercise with the certainty that you have intuitive awareness. You want to live; you need to eat to live. Rely on your intuition to determine the right foods and/or diet to live well.

Summary

Diets come and go; recipes succeed and fail; life goes on. Continuation is the thread that links your experiences together. With each experience, you have an opportunity to add to your growth. Each step along the path accumulates into intuitive awareness.

Lesson 26

Cornerstone

Make whole grains a cornerstone of your diet.

A cornerstone is the first stone set in the construction of a masonry foundation; it is vitally important because all other stones are set in reference to this stone. Today, we use the word cornerstone to mean a basic element, a foundation, a focus.

When you organize your meal planning or design your diet, it is important to have a foundation with a focus on health. There are a number of reasons why whole grains are ideal as the cornerstone of this foundation:

1. The majority of people around the world rely on grains as the basis of their diet, from the peoples of Asia who consume rice to the peoples of Latin America who eat corn to the peoples of Europe who consume bread. One of my friends from Belgium feels that meals are incomplete without naturally-leavened bread; one of my Japanese friends feels the same way about rice.

2. The growth of whole grains coincided with human evolution. For example, there were no grains during the age of dinosaurs or the age of developing mammals. Rather, grains came into existence with the growth of modern-day humans. It is speculated that grains helped homo sapiens develop the large brain that set our species apart! Since the agricultural revolution, humans have cultivated whole

grains, and civilizations have continued to expand and flourish.

3. Whole grains have the capacity to feed entire populations. Ecologically, grains produce more nutrition per acre than meat. Economically, grains cost less than meat when feeding the same number of people. Nutritionally, whole grains provide more density and complex carbohydrates than fruits. Practically, whole grains can be easily stored for long periods of time unlike meat or starchy vegetables, which spoil relatively quickly.

4. Whole grains have a prominent place in the world market. They are easily shipped between countries for everyday supply, particularly in times of relief.

5. Grains have status in language and myth. The word *meal* is derived from the Latin word "mele," which means grain. Meal also means "measure," as in to measure grain. Myths about grains are present in every culture, with tales of the gods bestowing grains on people or of abundant harvests being assured by certain deities. Festivals and songs evolved to celebrate this plentitude, and they endure in such events as our tradition of Thanksgiving. Grains were and are revered as the sustenance of life.

6. Whole grains are delicious, and they can be fashioned into countless foods. Their flavors stem from complex carbohydrates that convert slowly to glucose, which we enjoy as the satisfying taste of sweetness and which sustains us over significant periods of time.

Cornerstone, like continuation, is a concept that can be applied to food and our relationship with food.

Exercise 26: Whole Grain as Cornerstone

Throughout recorded history, many people around the world depended on whole cereal grains as their main food, the cornerstone of their diet. The *Cultural Menus* in *Appendix 5* list various countries and their local grains.

For today, consume a whole grain at one of your meals; it need not be the majority of the meal. At the same time, consider what it would mean to make whole grains the cornerstone of your diet.

Summary

Grains are a cornerstone of human evolution and, historically, have been integral to humankind's diet. If you make grain a cornerstone of your meals, you will experience benefits to your body, mind, spirit, and intuition.

Lesson 27

Life Force 1: Whole Grains

Life force is the power that creates and continues life.
It is both the activity of life and the potential of life.
Life force ensures life continues.

Life force is a mystery. Think of a seed…a small hard round thing, seemingly lifeless. But, add water and it changes. It absorbs moisture, the outer shell cracks, and a sprout shoots out. If planted, the sprout will send down roots, grow a stalk, mature, flower, and produce seeds. The cycle of life continues.

You, yourself, live thanks to your own life force. You tap into it when eating because all foods have life force. For today, consider the life force in whole grains. Do you know that a kernel of grain can sprout after millennia due to its tremendous life force? It has been documented that some grains of spelt and kamut, found in tombs in Egyptian pyramids, sprouted when soaked, even after lying dormant for thousands of years!

We can observe this life force in a kernel of grain, which contains an outer hull (the bran) and an internal part (the endosperm—the starchy part of the grain that contains the carbohydrates). Also present inside the kernel is the germ, which contains the fat of the kernel and is the place from which the grain sprouts. When a kernel sprouts, it produces a tiny living plant inside the endosperm. When large enough, the burgeoning plant pushes through the hull and sends out roots and a shoot.

As described, the life force of grain is present in the whole kernel. Thus, when grains are refined and the hull and germ are removed, the grain loses its vitality, B vitamins, fiber (concentrated nutrition found in the hull), and Vitamin E (found in the germ). It is significant that a refined grain, having lost its life force, cannot sprout. Clearly, this has implications for the nutritive aspect of grains.

Therefore, whole grains are recommended because they contain full nutrition as nature intended. They have nourished humankind for thousands of years, being the food of our ancestors. Also, they are universal, able to easily feed people around the globe and curb malnutrition and associated poverty. My favorite reason for recommending whole grains is their tremendous life force, the capacity to nourish and sustain life nutritionally, the ability to start new plants and new life.

Exercise 27: The Life Force of Grains

Experience the life force in brown rice by soaking it for 2 to 3 hours before cooking. Use the same measurements, the same pan, and the same timing as other times you cooked brown rice. This time, when eating the rice, chew the first mouthful as long as possible, allowing your saliva to mingle with the grain. Does it taste different from grain that wasn't soaked? I have found I can extract a considerable amount of sweetness using this method of cooking and eating.

Here is information on the benefits of soaking grains:

1. Soaking helps the grain cook more evenly. Grains are the

seeds of the plant, which are dried to remove moisture before storage. Soaking before cooking allows the grain to reabsorb water, causing the inner endosperm of the kernels to become plump. When cooking, the heat more easily penetrates to the interior of the kernel, helping the grain to cook more thoroughly. This process requires about the same amount of time as cooking without soaking, but the texture and taste can be slightly different.

2. Soaking improves digestion. Grains possess an amazing capacity for long storage due to enzyme inhibitors and phytates that prevent them from decomposing. This factor is highly valuable when you need a bag of rice to last through the winter. These inhibitors and phytates are not so good for your digestive system. Soaking neutralizes them.

3. Soaking activates the life force of the grain. Because soaking activates enzymes and carbohydrates, it is the first step in sprouting grains. If rice (or another grain) is soaked for 24 hours, drained, then repeatedly soaked, rinsed, and drained, the kernel will sprout. While 24 hours is not enough time for a fully developed sprout to form, it is enough time for the grain to swell and activate its life force, making it highly desirable for consumption.

Summary

For centuries, grains have supplied life force for countless numbers of people, especially when soaked and cooked properly. Use your intuition to recognize the life force in grains and how best to utilize it to support your own life force.

Note: All sprouted foods contain life force. Fully developed sprouts are used in many products from breads to supplements. For information on growing sprouts yourself, refer to *Appendix 5.*

Lesson 28

Life Force 2: Fermented Foods

*Life force is the power of life itself. While
we can be aware of it at any point, it shows
up vibrantly at birth and at death.*

We can observe life force at a baby's birth or at someone's passing, times of tremendous energy and importance. Witnesses report awe and respect; if you have ever been present at a birth or a passing, you know it is an amazing event.

We also can see life force in food. It is present in the soaking and sprouting process and in the fermentation process. Fermentation changes food due to the action of microbes. Microbes break down substances; in that, they are agents of "death." They are also agents of "life" as they release natural sugars that add deliciousness and rich flavor to foods. Microbes are beneficial agents that connect the cycle of death and birth and ensure the continuation of the life cycle.

Fermentation is simply allowing ingredients to rest (in appropriate conditions) for a period before being consumed. In time, the food changes to a new product. Some fermented foods are wine, cheese, pickles, yogurt, miso, naturally-leavened breads, beer, sausages, vinegars, and soy sauce. Fermented products are common to all civilizations and are consumed alongside grains, often on a daily basis.

Traditional peoples discovered that fermenting food made a difference. For example, a clean and pure source of water wasn't always available, so water was combined with other ingredients and fermented to produce beer and wine for consumption. Yogurt and cultured milk products kept longer than fresh milk. Cheese could keep over a long winter. Naturally-leavened bread was lighter than unleavened bread. In India, dhal (beans) were soaked and allowed to slightly ferment before being eaten. In Europe, people made sauerkraut. The Japanese developed miso, umeboshi plums, and soy sauce. Different locales are famous for their wine, cheese, or miso. The culinary techniques developed to make these foods have become an art form, and these techniques are still in use today.

Fermented foods are more than mere commodities; these foods enhance health. They provide lactic acid, which adds beneficial bacteria (microbes) to the intestinal tract and strengthens the flora, leading to better digestion and assimilation by your body. When eaten at the same time as beans and grains, fermented foods help neutralize phytates that interfere with good digestion. Other fermented foods soothe the stomach, aiding the natural secretion of hydrochloric acid. Not surprisingly, fermented foods have been revered and respected through human history as a way to improve health.

Exercise 28: The Life Force of Fermented Foods

Consume a naturally fermented food with your grain, at one meal or more. Pickles complement grains well, such as eating sauerkraut with bread or kimchi with rice. Miso soup also accompanies meals well and it helps the entire body. Chew well, savor the flavors, and receive the benefits from eating these foods at the same meal. For more information on fermented foods, see *Appendix 5*.

Summary

Fermented foods are one of the secrets of healthy eating and are used to balance meals, enhance health, and increase physical vitality. These benefits lead to stronger intuition, which, in turn, helps you discern quality fermented foods.

Note: If you are sensitive to molds or have candida, you may need to consult a health care practitioner about the advisability of consuming fermented products. If you are unable to eat fermented foods, make a special effort to consciously increase your saliva production. Saliva breaks down carbohydrates in the mouth and begins the digestion process. While it is not a pickle, it can greatly enhance your sense of well-being.

Lesson 29

Food Combining

Food combining is using the energy of foods, more than one at a time, for optimum benefit.

Think of things you would never eat together. Now, think of all the things you love to eat at the same time. That's food combining. Most people practice some sort of food combining, such as a gourmet chef designing a menu or a picky eater choosing one thing over another.

Food combining theories are based on the mechanisms of digestion. The human digestive tract is composed of three main areas—mouth, stomach, and small intestine—with different digestive juices in each area. Saliva, the digestive juice in the mouth, contains amylase, an enzyme that works on the digestion of starches (carbohydrates). Gastric juice works on food in the stomach; it is composed of different enzymes, based on the particular food. Protein requires pepsin, and fats need lipase.

The ideal situation occurs when these enzymes work one at a time, or, if together, they complement each other. When enzymes conflict, the groupings don't digest as well. For example, pepsin works on protein and is highly acidic. Amylase digests carbohydrates; it is neutralized in a highly acidic environment. While whole grains and beans combine and digest well, fruits and beans don't. Fruit and animal foods don't either, nor do carbohydrates and animal foods.

In addition to proper combinations, proper timing is important. Some foods digest faster than others. For example, melons digest in 20 to 30 minutes, raw fruits in 1 hour, and complex carbohydrates in 2 to 3 hours. So, eating a melon with apples or a sandwich with a banana are less-than-ideal combinations. Food-combining suggestions are especially useful in times of poor digestion or sickness. Most people eat simple foods when sick, choosing one or two foods and eating them without elaborate preparation.

Food-combining ideas further the specifics about nutrition and are useful in determining what assimilates well together. If you have a delicate digestion or any digestive problems, try some of these ideas and use your intuition to determine the benefit:

1. Eat melons solo. Melons digest more quickly than any other food, even other fruits, and your stomach processes them best alone.

2. Eat cooked grains and raw fruits separately, especially citrus fruits. Oranges, grapefruits, and other citrus are more acidic than grains; the acids destroy amylase, thus interfering with the digestion of carbohydrates. Small amounts of lemon juice are an exception. For example, salad with a dressing that includes lemon juice served alongside a sandwich is easier to digest than a glass of orange juice and the sandwich.

3. Avoid eating beans and fruit together. Each requires different digestive juices; neither digests well when consumed together. For years, I have told my kids that this combo produces farts! As teenagers, they still practice this rule (most of the time). However, if there are times when it can't be avoided, wait at least 15 minutes after eating beans before having dessert or juice.

4. For ongoing digestive troubles, consider simplifying your meals, eating proteins and carbohydrates at different times of the day. Eat breakfast with one or two compatible items;

lunch with a protein and salad (such as beans, tofu, or chicken with a salad or other vegetables); and dinner with rice and vegetables. Although this may sound at odds with previous information in this book, consider this information as refinement—satisfying your nutritional needs of carbohydrate, protein, and fat throughout the day.

5. Pay attention to cookbooks and dietary manuals that recommend certain combinations. Some herbs enhance digestion as do sea vegetables.

6. Simplify your diet in the case of food allergies. A rotation diet to reduce food allergies respects many food-combining principles.

7. Consume fermented foods (pickles) with grains. Of all the combinations I have encountered over the years, this universally practiced one is highly valuable. Japanese people eat rice with miso soup and pickles; Germans eat dark bread and sauerkraut; people in India eat rice, fermented beans (dhal), and/or chutneys (fermented fruits). Many condiments, from salsa to kimchi to yogurt, are examples of culinary staples that are traditionally fermented and consumed alongside grains.

Exercise 29: Food Combinations

Make a list of foods you avoid because you don't like how they taste together or they make your stomach hurt, give you gas or diarrhea. Now, make a list of combinations that you love to eat together and that sit well in your stomach. These lists are references for your own personal food combination needs and originate from your intuitive awareness of what agrees with you and what doesn't.

Summary

Everyone loves potlucks and buffets, yet who likes them at every meal? Or even every day? Food combining can help you feel better because it is a way to simplify. Eating and preparing food need not be difficult, long, or a cause to hurt your stomach. Follow basic guidelines to help yourself intuitively—and pay attention: sometimes your intuition tells you to eat everything! Other times intuition tells you to eat one thing at a time. Food-combining rules are one method to help you sort it out. Let the food you eat at the same time nourish you and your intuition.

Lesson 30

REVIEW: **Principles: The Framework of Diet**

Savor the flavor.

In this unit, you learned some principles for diet beyond simple nutrition. These principles strengthen and stabilize your health and further your intuitive awareness.

Review what you learned using the following summary of lessons:

Lesson 25: Continuation. This guiding principle recognizes your past and anticipates your future through celebrating your strength. The lesson focused on grains as an example of continuity and reviewed your personal evolution of dietary consciousness.

Lesson 26: Cornerstone. This second principle focused on whole grain as a cornerstone of diet. Throughout history, whole grains nourished people as they do today.

Lessons 27 and 28: Life force. These two lessons talked about the principle of life force, the energy that keeps us alive, particularly noticeable at the beginning of life and the end of life. For foods, we see life force at the outset in the sprouting of foods and soaked grains. We again see life force in fermented food, the end product of the fermentation process.

Lesson 29: Food combining. This lesson emphasized the need of choosing complementary dishes with respect for digestion and avoiding combinations of food that cause unfavorable reactions.

Salt

This lesson continues with another important principle—salt and flavor. Salt is the universal seasoning agent with a very long history of use and respect. Evidence indicates that Neolithic people were boiling salt-laden spring water to extract salt as far back as 6050 BC. The word salary originates from Latin: salarium, which referred to the money paid to the Roman Army's soldiers for the purchase of salt. Gandhi evaporated salt from ocean water as part of his peaceful revolution for the people of India against the British monopoly on salt production and trade. Animals are drawn to saltlicks to satisfy their need for this substance. There are other reasons for the importance of salt:

1. *Flavor*. Food cooked with salt is more flavorful than without. Salt brings out the delicious flavor of foods and heightens the flavors of other herbs and spices.

2. *Cooking*. Grains require a bit of salt to cook thoroughly. Salt added to beans (after the beans have been fully cooked) helps reduce gas.

3. *Nutrient source*. Salt provides sodium and chlorine, two minerals needed by the body. Sodium and chlorine bind in the body with other minerals such as magnesium, phosphorous, and calcium. Together, these various combinations build bones and muscles and contribute to internal fluids.

4. *Digestion*. Chlorine from salt combines with hydrogen in

water and contributes to hydrochloric acid, a gastric acid used by the stomach for digestion. In addition, when salt crystals are cooked into food, they become surrounded and buffered by other molecules to ease transition into the body.

5. *Balance*. Salt adds an alkaline-forming factor to all foods, especially grains. It helps the body maintain a slightly alkaline condition and works to balance the acid-forming quality of grain. In disease prevention, salt can be a helpful component. Sodium is one of the primary electrolytes in the body. In fact, all four cationic electrolytes (sodium, potassium, magnesium, and calcium) are available in unrefined salt, as are other vital minerals needed for optimal bodily function.

6. *Sufficient quantity*. Salt is not present in large quantities in fresh foods. If you prepare all your own food, you need some salt for flavor, balance, and to avoid deficiency. If you don't use salt over a long time, you can become deficient in sodium. Sometimes people adopt a low-salt diet for health reasons. If this is your situation, realize you can reduce your salt intake by limiting or avoiding most packaged and restaurant foods (they usually contain high amounts of salt). Another way to control your intake of salt is by cooking your own food.

7. *Fermentation*. Many microorganisms cannot live in an overly salty environment: water is drawn out of their cells by osmosis. For this reason salt is used to ferment some foods, such as vegetables, and to preserve others, such as smoked bacon or fish.

Exercise 30-1: Flavors in Cuisines

It is one thing to appreciate simple fare and another to subsist on it. Most people want flavor in their meals. But "simple" need not be boring and it doesn't mean eating only one thing. Grains are often perceived as boring; however, they are rarely eaten alone. We put butter on bread or sauce on pasta. It is normal to want flavor in food. Few people choose plain food unless they are sick, have stomach problems, or are frail. While infants and children often prefer mild food, most adults prefer more flavor.

For this exercise, observe what foods various cuisines serve together. What are the dishes that accompany grains? You can look at the *Cultural Menus* in this book, read cookbooks, or recall what you ate at a restaurant or while traveling. Chances are that you will see that grains are simple (sometimes bland or neutral) but are served with foods that contain a wealth of flavors: sauces, chutneys, beans, and condiments. Many times, other dishes are the main course and the rice or other grain is merely a side dish.

Exercise 30-2: Try a New Recipe to Accompany a Grain

Prepare a new recipe (for you) today to serve with your grains. See *Appendix 5* or your favorite cookbook for recipes.

Summary

Use principles in determining what to eat. Grain is a continuation factor in building a healthy diet. Cook it with a little salt and include flavorful foods and fermented vegetables. Let it be a cornerstone of your meals, your health, and your intuition. Take care of yourself and let your intuition flourish.

Note: The salt test in *Appendix 3* helps you intuitively determine good-quality salt.

NEW PARADIGM

There is a connection between body and spirit.

In this unit, you learn about the connection between body and spirit and the role of this connection in healing. You learn about the importance of blood and that a change in diet causes a change in blood, which can precipitate a paradigm shift—a change in perception.

Keyword: Healing

The body has the capacity to remember and return to what is important, whether physical healing or spiritual renewal. When a person makes a change in diet, there is an opportunity for physical healing. Because body and spirit are connected, when you nourish one, you nurture the other. Thus, physical healing renews the spirit, and you can use your intuition in nourishing and nurturing both.

Food: Continue to Eat Healthy Food

Build on what you know to be appropriate for yourself and incorporate ideas from this course as applicable.

Exercise: Plan Menus

Use these steps to plan menus and to coordinate with the lessons:

1. Use the *Life Template* and *Menu Template* from Lesson 7 to organize your time and to chart menus.

2. For lessons 31 to 35, plan menus to fit your needs.

3. For lesson 36, include a healthy dessert.

4. Consult any menus from *Appendix 5* and *Appendix 6* as desired.

Resources: Appendix 6
◊ *Intuition about sweeteners and desserts*
◊ *Food Combining Menus*
◊ *Discharge*

Getting Started: Lessons 31 to 36

Everyone has an idea about the meaning of healing—a return to health in times of illness. In this unit, you learn about another aspect of healing—that healing the body strengthens the spirit.

Note: This unit expands into some of the emotional and mental aspects of intuition. Continue to rely on your intuition for feedback on what works for you.

Lesson 31

Blood

Blood is amazing...it does its work without fail and keeps us alive.

Blood is a necessity, continuously circulating to provide oxygen and nutrients to all parts of your body. Because blood is essential to your well-being, it is important to understand blood and how to take care of it.

Substance

Blood consists of red blood cells, white blood cells, platelets, and plasma, each of which has a defined role. An average adult body holds about five liters of blood.

Job

Red blood cells carry oxygen to your body. White blood cells are part of your immune system. Platelets help form clots. Plasma, the liquid part of blood, is mostly water and maintains normal hydration of tissues. It also transports all components of blood: cells, platelets, glucose, proteins, fats, vitamins, salts, and waste products of metabolism. Thus, blood delivers oxygen and nutrients to cells and tissues and, at the same time, transports carbon dioxide and metabolic byproducts to lungs and kidneys for elimination. These processes of renewal with oxygen and removal of waste repeat a million times every day. Blood is constantly circulating, day or night, in sickness or health, when active or quiet. When you are at rest, it takes about one minute for your heart to circulate the total volume of blood through your body.

Source

The average life cycle of a red blood cell is 120 days. Billions of red blood cells die off each day, and billions are produced by bone marrow to replace those that wear out and die. The spleen breaks down old red blood cells for disposal by the lungs.

Quality

"Blood quality" is a term that describes the health of the blood. Some qualities of blood are constant (such as blood type); other qualities can fluctuate (such as amount of fat suspended in the plasma). Many tests are available to determine various aspects of the blood. Blood health is affected by a number of factors ranging from diet to disease to the amount of pollution a person is exposed to.

Vital Essence

In traditional Chinese medicine, blood is considered one of the vital essences that provides life. Blood is life force; when blood is gone, life is gone. Blood is also linked with a person's spirit; when a person's spirit is gone, life is gone. Things that influence the vital essence of blood such as diet, environment, and ancestry also influence a person's spirit.

Diet

Diet has a direct affect on the quality of blood. Some things such as alcohol and white refined sugar affect blood right away. Alcohol impairs thinking, talking, and walking if the blood alcohol level is too high. White refined sugar enters the bloodstream immediately as glucose and produces a sugar high. Complex carbohydrates, on the other hand, provide glucose more slowly and feed the blood constantly, not causing extreme spikes. Proteins, fats, vitamins, and minerals also enter the bloodstream and are transported around the body. The quality and quantity of these nutrients affect the quality of your blood. For instance, poor-quality fats, especially an overabundance, accumulate over time, clog arteries, and lead to complications.

Healthy blood makes a healthy person. One of the most influential ways to improve the health of blood is to eat beneficial foods and to avoid harmful foods. When a person improves the diet, he or she can expect to feel better. A change in diet can affect the blood quality in as little as 10 days. Physical exercise is another way to improve the health of your blood.

Exercise 31-1: Pulse

This exercise makes you aware of your heart and blood. Do it once now and then again whenever you think of it to appreciate and enjoy your blood and body.

Find your pulse and count how many times your heart beats in one minute. Sit quietly, use the second hand on a clock, and count for one minute. Wiggle your fingers and toes and visualize your heart pulsing blood through your body with every beat. It takes only about one minute for blood to circulate once around the body.

To find your pulse, use the index and middle finger of one hand and place both at the wrist of the opposite arm or along one side of the neck. Search for a strong steady beat.

Exercise 31-2: Physical Movement

Physical exercise improves health. It increases heart rate, strengthens the heart muscle, and improves circulation. It also tones muscles and fortifies bones, which in turn increase bone marrow that produces red blood cells. Exercise can add years to your life. If you already exercise on a regular basis, continue engaging in these sports or activities.

If you do not exercise regularly, consider how to begin. Do some stretches, walk to the corner, or swing your arms and legs to music.

Today, take a short walk, ideally for 15 to 20 minutes, after your biggest meal of the day. Walking supports your digestion and increases your awareness of how much you ate. For instance, if you overeat, you probably won't feel like walking after eating. Instead, rise from the table after eating and proceed with a simple activity, such as washing dishes. As you move your body, notice how your stomach feels.

Summary

Intuition tells you that your heart takes care of you. It beats every second and circulates your blood continually. Be in awe of your heart and your blood and what they do to keep you healthy. In so doing, enhance your vitality and strengthen your intuition.

Lesson 32

Blood and Diet

*All types of diets have one thing in common:
they all strive to help a person thrive.*

Your blood is your lifeline. It is the fluid that circulates through your body carrying nutrients to and removing wastes from your cells. Your blood is vital to your life, and healthy blood is essential to your vitality.

What does it mean to have vitality? Vitality means to have energy, to feel strong, to be free from disease, and to have vibrancy throughout your life. You are able to do the things that make you happy. Vitality happens due to two factors—the inclusion of things that make you feel energized and the avoidance of things that deplete your energy. When you feel vital, you thrive.

Diet is particularly important in helping you thrive; the reason it is important is because what you eat affects the composition of your blood. Your diet affects your level of energy and vibrancy. Through digestion, the food you eat is broken down into glucose, amino acids, and lipids, the basic components of carbohydrates, proteins, and fats. When these components enter the bloodstream, they have the potential to do various things. Glucose reaches the cells and provides energy. Amino acids support the nervous system and provide building materials for muscle tissue and rejuvenation. Lipids aid the hormonal system, build cell walls, and store energy. Other nutrients from food also enter the bloodstream: vitamins, minerals, salt, as well as residues and chemicals present in your food. The foods that provide valuable substances are important, as covered in Unit 4—whole grains for complex carbohydrates, beans for plant-based proteins, and nuts and seeds for quality fats. It is also

Diet	Summary	Details
Vegetarian diet (no meat; dairy okay)	A vegetarian diet excludes meat, although eggs and dairy foods may be okay. High in complex carbohydrates, moderate in plant-based proteins, and moderate to low in fats.	Includes fruits, vegetables, nuts, seeds, oils, whole grains, and beans. Proportions vary by person according to individual needs: some vegetarians eat more fruits, others more vegetables, others more dairy, others more grains and beans.
Vegan diet (no animal foods)	A vegan diet excludes all animal products. High in carbohydrates, moderate in plant-based proteins, and moderate to low in fats.	Includes fruits, vegetables, nuts, seeds, oils, and whole grains and beans. Proportions vary by person according to individual needs.
Raw food diet (no cooking)	A raw food diet excludes all animal products and no heat is used in preparing food. Low in proteins and fats, high in carbohydrates.	Includes fruits and vegetables, sprouted grains and beans, and soaked nuts and seeds.
Paleo diet (caveman diet)	Named after Paleolithic humans, a paleo diet includes meat and no grains. High in animal proteins and fats; low in complex carbohydrates.	Includes meat, fish, eggs, nuts, seeds, and simple fruits and vegetables.
Atkins diet (high protein/low carb for weight loss)	Named after Dr. Robert C. Atkins, the Atkins diet includes meat and limited grains. High in animal proteins and fats, and low in carbohydrates.	Includes meat, fish, eggs, dairy foods, nuts, seeds, fruits, and vegetables. No refined grains are used although whole grains can be used in limited amounts.

Diet	Summary	Details
Macrobiotic diet (predominantly vegan, but may include some animal foods)	A macrobiotic approach emphasises whole foods. High in complex carbohydrates, moderate proteins, and low in fats.	Includes whole grains, beans, nuts, seeds, oils, vegetables, fruits, and sea vegetables. Some people are vegetarian; others eat fish and/or eggs.
Mediterranean diet (includes olive oil)	A Mediterranean diet includes whole foods and olive oil. High in complex carbohydrates, moderate proteins, moderate fats.	Includes whole grains, beans, nuts, seeds, fruits, vegetables, and olive oil. Animal foods and dairy foods are included.
Gluten-free diet (no gluten)	A gluten-free diet excludes all foods that contain gluten. Other foods are used as desired; proportions vary.	Only requirement is excluding gluten from the diet. Otherwise, this diet includes whatever the person desires.
Oil-free diet (no oil)	An oil-free diet is similar to a vegan diet in that it excludes animal fats and liquid vegetable oils in all preparations. High in complex carbohydrats, moderate in plant-based proteins, and low in fats.	Includes whole grain, beans, seeds, selected nuts, vegetables, and fruits.
Blood Type diet: Type A is more vegetarian, Type B is more dairy, Type AB is a mixture, Type O is more meat.	The Blood Type diet varies by blood type. For example, people with Blood Type O can eat more animal protein than people with blood type A. Proportions vary.	Includes animal foods, grains, beans, nuts, seeds, vegetables, fruits, and oils for specific Blood Type. Wheat is not recommended for any blood type.

important to avoid refined foods, foods high in pesticide residue, and food containing additives.

There are many popular diets today. They are often divided into two camps—those that include meat and animal products and those that avoid animal products. When you review the literature, most explain why to follow one diet or another. Oftentimes, the explanations are based on how these foods affect the blood. While there is general agreement among most diets about the desirability of avoiding refined carbohydrates and eating plenty of vegetables, there are diverging opinions and scientific data concerning fats and proteins and what sources are best.

Medical physicians John McDougall, Dean Ornish, Neil Barnard, and Caldwell Esselstyn propose a complete vegetarian diet for their clients who suffer from heart disease. They also stress abstinence from fats in not only animal foods but in liquid oils. The scientific data say that diets high in fat and cholesterol cause fat levels in blood to rise, which in turn can lead to heart disease. Each doctor recommends avoiding animal foods—meat, eggs, fish, and dairy—because these foods contain high amounts of fats. They have worked with innumerable patients who have had considerable success with their recommendations. Dr. Andrew Weil agrees with such restrictions for someone with chronic disease. For someone in relatively good health, he recommends a Mediterranean diet that includes olive oil and adequate essential fatty acids. He encourages people to eat a modified vegetarian diet, where one eats mostly plant-based proteins. Another physician, Dr. Gabriel Cousins, recommends a raw food vegetarian diet for his patients. His plan includes plenty of fruits, vegetables, sprouted grains and beans, and essential fatty acids from flax or coconut oil.

On the other side are authorities such as Robert Atkins, M.D. and Weston Price, D.D.S., who both recommend inclusion of animal proteins in the diet. Specifically, Atkins advocates a diet for weight loss that is low in carbohydrates and high in animal protein. He postulates that carbohydrates, especially when refined, contribute to obesity, insulin demands, and diabetes. Weston Price, a dentist who has traveled extensively and observed a number of traditional cultures, searched for groups of people untouched by civilization who were in vibrant health and free from disease and dental decay. He observed that they ate a diet that included whole foods, plant-based proteins, and modest amounts of animal foods. Diets based on Weston Price's teachings stress including high-quality animal food along with whole grains, beans, seeds, nuts, and plenty of vegetables. His proponents advocate this diet particularly for children and women of child-bearing age.

Another variation is the "Blood Type Diet" proposed by naturopath Peter D'Adamo. Dr. D'Adamo theorizes that different blood types react to food differently; therefore, he recommends various refinements for each blood type. Blood Type O, for instance, benefits from including animal protein on a regular basis, while Blood Type A thrives on little, if any, animal protein. Macrobiotic practitioners also recommend adaptations for people based on their varying needs. Overall, macrobiotics stresses whole foods and plant-based proteins, adding animal proteins for certain people in certain situations.

Everyone wants to thrive; each of these diets was developed in an attempt to help people thrive. Some are recommended to remove obstacles to thriving; others include suggestions to ensure thriving. Everybody has a unique set of circumstances in which to thrive; what helps one person thrive may not help another. Perhaps you have met a vegetarian who is energetic or another vegetarian who is pale and weak. You may know someone who thrives on animal foods and another consumer of animal foods who has health problems. Learning what makes you thrive involves paying attention and relying on your intuition for feedback on what does and doesn't work for you. Paying attention to your intuition helps you learn what helps you thrive. This is the key.

Exercise 32: Diets and Thriving

Read the descriptions of diets in this lesson and determine whether you (or anyone you know) have used or are using any of them. Consider whether the diet is helping you thrive; if it is, reflect on why you are thriving. Perhaps it is because you are excluding something, or including something, or have changed the proportion of nutrients. If you haven't used any of these diets, think about others you have used.

Summary

Intuitively, we want to thrive. Accordingly, we seek those foods that help us thrive. Let your intuition help you identify the foods that benefit you the most so you can thrive in your physical body and in your acceptance of others and their needs.

Lesson 33

Blood and Healing

Blood has the ability to heal.

Blood is miraculous—it rejuvenates and heals. Food is very important in rejuvenation because the quality of your food determines the quality of your blood. If your food is free of excess toxins, your blood is free of excess toxins, and your cells have a better environment in which to reproduce. When your diet changes to foods that include fewer toxins, your blood responds positively. Little by little, your blood removes old toxins and cleanses faster due to healthier nourishment with fewer burdens. While it takes about four months for a complete overhaul of your total blood volume, enough blood cells can change in as few as ten days for you to notice a difference. Over time, other cells in the body begin to change too. As cells replicate in healthier blood, they begin to detox or discharge excess toxins and other unwanted materials. When blood is healthy, cells receive the right nourishment so they can replicate without excess stress.

The body's rejuvenation process, starting with cellular reproduction, is nothing less than a miracle. Cells constantly and automatically divide, making exact copies with the same DNA and other cellular information. In addition to replication, cells also constantly die and are replaced by new cells as another part of rejuvenation and healing. We see this process externally in nail and hair growth and in the shedding of outer skin layers after sunburn. The inside of the body changes too, some parts more quickly than others. Stomach lining cells are replaced every five to ten days; highly acidic gastric juices cause them to wear out quickly. Liver cells, on the other hand, may take years to rejuvenate. As noted before, blood cells for the total volume of blood renew over a period of about four months. Because new cells are constantly being created, the body always has a chance to heal and reinvent itself.

One important part of healing is the blood's ability to clot. When my son had his wisdom teeth extracted, the dentist told us how to monitor the healing. He said the blood clot that forms over the extraction is more than a covering to close the gap and prevent infection. The blood clot lays the foundation for new tissue to develop. Furthermore, if the blood clot is displaced, the body cannot produce another one, and the wound will not heal properly. Needless to say, my son took good care of his mouth. And both of us developed a new appreciation for blood.

Clearly, your overall health depends on the quality of your blood. With high-quality blood, your health improves, your mind clears, and your emotions stabilize. Your spirit is also affected; you have a chance to be happier. Healing arises due to all of these components, both physical improvement and spiritual enhancement. *Change diet; change blood; change cells; change yourself.*

Exercise 33: Evaluate Energy Level

The limited one-day fast in Lesson 16 included advice to continue consuming more vegetal quality foods and abstain from red meats, dairy foods, and junk foods as much as possible. For today, the exercise is to evaluate your energy level. How do you feel since the fast in Lesson 16? Do you feel better than before? The same? Worse? Be as honest as you can. Many people have a positive reaction to the elimination of dairy, meat, and junk foods. But this doesn't mean if you feel the same, or worse, that you are doing something wrong. Consciously striving to take care of yourself is always right.

Summary

Blood powers rejuvenation, which is facilitated by avoiding negative substances and enhancing positive ones. A change in diet affects the quality of your blood and its rejuvenating ability. Intuitively, we know to take care of ourselves. When we take care of what we eat and drink, we take care of our blood, and in turn our blood continues to take care of us.

Note: Healing can involve detox and/or discharge. See *Appendix 6* for information.

Lesson 34

The Big Picture

What does your spirit want?

Everyone wants to be healthy; everyone wants to be strong. We all want fulfilling relationships, a satisfying career, and happy children. Each of us creates many goals during our lifetime. The "big picture" refers to our overall life's goal—the major contributions that matter most and the people we love unconditionally.

Often a person on his or her deathbed reviews the "big picture" of their life, remembering things done and undone as they reflect on career, family, and sense of purpose. We can use a similar reflection of the "big picture" in any difficult situation.

When my first son was born, I vowed to feed him as healthily as possible. I ate a strict vegan macrobiotic diet with no animal or dairy foods. When my second son was born, I became ill, and by the time he was six months old, he was ill too. I later found out I was deficient in Vitamin B_{12}. The doctor diagnosed the baby as "failure to thrive" and recommended adding dairy and animal foods to his diet.

This was a difficult decision for me. It broke my heart to think I had done something to hurt him. But I struggled with the idea of feeding cheese, yogurt, and chicken to a young child because I saw these foods as not part of a healthy diet. The idea that helped most was to consider the big picture. Above all, I wanted him to be healthy. So, I chose what he needed over my preconceived notions about dairy and animal products.

I bought yogurt and cottage cheese and served it with his rice and vegetables. I prepared chicken soup for the first time in my life. I took B_{12} supplements and gave them to him too. He regained his strength and now, after many years, you would never know he had been ill as a baby.

This experience changed my attitude about diet. Before I knew about my vitamin B_{12} deficiency, I had an idealized concept about diet. After this experience, I learned to be practical. Raising children initiated tremendous personal growth; many times, I had to look further than my own ideals. Through the years, other events came up where I had to decide between ideal or practical. Pepperoni pizza, birthday parties, fast food, soda, beer…the list goes on and on. My decision was not so much whether I should be flexible or engage in battle, but to focus on loving my kids for who they are and still stay committed to the "big picture" of helping each of them grow into a loving, responsible adult, fully equipped to make decisions about food (and other things) amidst the changing circumstances of life.

Exercise 34: Consider Life in Future

Look at your goals. Where do you want to be—healthwise—in 10 years? By the time you die? Do you desire freedom from pain? More flexibility? Do you think you will be different? How? Then, look at your "big picture." Do you desire fulfillment in your career, ease in your relationships with your family, inner peace?

Your answers to these questions may be similar to the goals you set in Lesson 18. If so, recognize the recurring theme(s). Whether your answers are the same or new, use this information and your intuitive sense to reveal your "big picture"—what your spirit desires.

Summary

Your spirit wants to engage in life fully. Choose to live in ways that support your long-term goals. Let your intuition influence your choices. This method honors intuition—the force that unites body and spirit.

Lesson 35

Nourishing Your Spirit

What is your spirit hungry for?

Your spirit is hungry for nourishment and nurturing. In Lesson 34, we concentrated on your "big picture"—what your spirit wants. In this lesson, we concentrate on foods that feed your spirit. These foods can be those served at celebrations such as a Thanksgiving meal or a birthday party. They may be foods avoided during religious holidays, such as Passover Seder, Ramadan, or Lent, or served during religious rites such as bread, representing the body of Christ in some sects of Christianity or Challah, a symbol of divine presence for Shabbat (the Sabbath) in Judaism. They also may be foods associated with certain events, such as the first tomato from the summer garden.

These foods nourish the spirit because they provide a bond with other people, hold significance from a belief system, and give us a connection to nature. We need meaningful events in our lives, and food often plays a role, sometimes the central role, in representing the meaning of the occasion.

My husband, Carl, and I maintain a tradition that nourishes our family. Carl grew up with the custom of a smorgasbord each Christmas Eve, a Swedish tradition that includes Swedish meatballs, lutefisk (a dried strong-flavored fish), cheeses, and crackers. We celebrate this tradition every year in our immediate family, serving organic cheeses, crackers made with natural ingredients, and seitan cutlets (wheat gluten also known as wheat meat) instead of meatballs. Sometimes we have fish, but, over the years, our smorgasbord has evolved to include items such as tofu, chips and guacamole, or roasted almonds. Very rarely do we spend the holiday with extended family as we live too far apart. However, the year we did, we were treated to a more traditional smorgasbord with Swedish meatballs. It was a true nourishment of spirit to dine with family for the holidays and eat the traditional fare—another example of choosing to eat in accordance with the "big picture" rather than "ideal" dietary principles.

It is good to participate in events that offer value to our lives. Today, the exercises elaborate on how to feed your spirit.

Exercise 35-1: Foods that Nourish the Spirit

Think of one event, which includes food, that nourishes your spirit. Examples include parties, celebrations, cultural events, religious holidays, or once-in-a-lifetime events such as weddings. Recall the foods that are served and then consider how you cherish these foods that are linked to the event. Maybe these foods are symbolic, such as the bitter herbs for Seder. Or maybe the dish is a recipe handed down through generations. We also cherish items that are expensive, exotic, or unique, as for a cultural festival.

Exercise 35-2: Food and Attitude

Food nourishes the body; when your body is nourished, so is your spirit. When your spirit is nourished, your body responds in a positive way. This exercise elaborates on two responses to food—

positive (happy) and negative (sad). Think of foods such as birthday cake, Passover Seder, Christmas smorgasbord, or recipes from grandma that make you smile. Now, think of foods that carry a negative connotation. These foods may include overcooked vegetables, foods you were forced to eat when you were young, foods you've eaten to lose weight, or foods you've eaten in the hope of recovering from a disease such as cancer.

Happy and sad are attitudes about food—one nourishes the spirit; the other doesn't. To really nourish your spirit, consider foods that make you really happy. It's not just about taste, or pleasure, or associations. But happy. Happy food. Of course, it helps if food is healthy too.

Exercise 35-3: Food, Spirit, and Healing

When happy and healthy are combined, you have the best of both worlds—foods that help your body and foods that help your spirit. This is the prerequisite for healing. For this exercise, write down the healthy foods that make you happy. Notice how you feel as you generate this list.

Summary

Food and spirituality are rarely combined in the same sentence. Yet, your spirit is with you every day and, like your body, needs nurturing every day. Let food feed your spirit. Let your intuition help you identify what it is that you love and let this be the determining factor. Feed your spirit and nourish your body. Feed your body and nourish your spirit.

Lesson 36

REVIEW: **New Paradigm**

Nourish the body to nurture the spirit.
Nourish the spirit to nurture the body.

The theme for this unit is that there is a connection between body and spirit. The new paradigm is to acknowledge this connection and use it to heal.

Food has the power to heal body and spirit. The lessons in this unit delved into this power by discussing food and how a change in diet affects your blood, health, and spirit. This lesson recaps the details and culminates in a practical exercise about healing: namely, to make a dessert that will nourish both your body and your spirit.

Here are summaries of the lessons:

Lesson 31: Blood. Blood is the substance of life and vitality, and the health of the blood affects the health of the person.

Lesson 32: Blood and diet. Your diet affects your blood, and is a determining factor in helping you thrive.

Lesson 33: Blood and healing. Blood heals and renews a person. A change in diet can change the healing power of blood in a short time.

Lesson 34: The big picture. What does your spirit desire? Your spirit wants to engage in life fully. Accessing your big picture can help during difficult times.

Lesson 35: Nourishing your spirit. What is your spirit hungry for? There are foods that nourish your spirit and that bring you happiness.

Today, celebrate the fact that you are nourishing your spirit when you nurture your body and that you are nourishing your body when you nurture your spirit. The following exercises elaborate on this concept.

Exercise 36-1: Make a Healthy Dessert

Healthy desserts nourish body and spirit simultaneously. Desserts can provide spiritual nourishment because they lift you up and help you feel relaxed, content, and happy. Desserts say, "Celebrate!" Prepare a recipe of your choice, simple or elaborate, and use only healthy ingredients. Use the *Intuition about Desserts* resource (*Appendix 6*), as needed. When you eat, notice how much you enjoy it.

Exercise 36-2: Tips for Navigating Social Events

Social events often are celebrations with abundant foods and desserts. There are other healthy and nurturing aspects such as getting together with friends. There also are, or can be, unhealthy aspects such as excessive alcohol, cake with high-fat, sugar frosting, or dishes made with ingredients you find unhealthy.

There is a time to feed the body and a time to feed the spirit. Ideally, you do both all the time. However, if social events present a conflict, I suggest you feed your spirit unless the consequences are too grave, such as a peanut allergy. Here are tips for keeping happy events healthy:

1. Focus on the reason for the event. Let the celebration nourish your spirit. Food is secondary.

2. Eat something before the event, especially if there will be foods you don't want to eat. Don't arrive feeling as though you're "starving." At the very least, drink a large glass of water before you go.

3. Be firm about what you won't put into your mouth. For me, it is fast food, candy, and sugary desserts from mass-produced facilities. I feel awful from sugar, so it is not worth eating it. However, if someone bakes something from

scratch, I often take a small piece because I enjoy personal creations. At these times, I pay attention to my reaction.

4. Choose the healthiest food and drinks possible. Carry a glass of water or tea around with you. Participate in the event without drawing attention to the items you are not eating.

5. Fill your plate with grapes or raw vegetables and a small amount of dip.

6. Go through the food line last. If a sit-down meal, eat more slowly than everyone else.

7. Focus on being with people rather than on eating food. Be interested in the company.

8. Bring a dish. Share healthy and happy food, whether dessert, entrée, or salad.

9. Initiate a new tradition, such as sushi for a Christmas party or seitan in place of meatballs.

10. Do other things. Dance, serve food to others, help the host, or clean up.

11. Leave before the last person.

12. Drink in moderation, if at all. Be safe.

13. Thank the host.

Summary

The body and spirit are not separate. They are connected. They affect each other. When we do things that affect the body, we affect the spirit. When we do things that affect the spirit, we affect the body. Let intuition help you eat nourishing foods, and in doing so, recognize you are nurturing your spirit. Also, let intuition guide you to nourish your spirit, and in so doing, nurture your body. Let intuition be the connection, the unifying force.

Taking Care of Yourself

*Recognize that it is wise to love yourself, to appreciate
who you are—right now—and to acknowledge that you
do the right things in the best way possible.*

In this unit, you reflect on your many assets, and you evaluate how
you take care of yourself. In the process, you become more aware
of how your spirit and body interact; you learn how to access your
inner wisdom. Ultimately, you recognize that this wisdom comes
from the love you have for yourself, not as self-importance, but as
kindness and gentleness for who you are.

Keyword: Love

Love is an attitude that applies to how you behave and how you
think. It affects both how you interact with other people and how
you relate to food. The objective of this unit is to recognize that love
is present in your life because you take care of yourself. Notice the
love in various areas of your life and use your intuition to increase it.

Food: Incorporate Skills

For this unit, eat healthy, nutritious food and incorporate skills
already acquired.

Exercise: Plan Menus

For this unit, use the following suggestions as appropriate:

1. Use the *Life Template* and *Menu Template* from Lesson 7 to schedule time and plan menus.

2. Consult any menus from the appendices, as desired.

3. Lesson 37 discusses a healthy bedroom. For this day, finish your last meal two to three hours before bedtime so you digest your food before sleeping.

4. Lesson 38 introduces a discussion on the world of opposites. Prepare a meal with some contrasts, whatever that means to you.

5. Lessons 39, 40, and 41 flow from one to the next. One exercise is used for all three lessons but from differing points of view. If possible, have meals for these three days flow into one another. See *Intuition about Leftovers* in *Appendix 7*.

6. Lesson 42 is the review lesson and talks about the Absence of Conflict. Prepare what you want or go out to eat. See *Intuition about Restaurants* in *Appendix 7*.

Resources: Appendix 7
◊ *Intuition about Leftovers*
◊ *Intuition about Eating Out*

Getting Started: Lessons 37 to 42
Everyone has a vested interest in his or her own well-being. Everyone wants to have enough to eat, adequate clothing, and a place to sleep. This unit covers various ways you take care of yourself and how your intuition influences your choices.

Note: Many self-help manuals talk about changing "this or that" because "such and such" is harmful. Avoid this type of thinking. The intent of this course is one of honoring your strengths, not of pointing out your weaknesses. As you progress through this unit, reflect on how you do the right things in the best way possible. Recognize that intuition is present within you. As you build a strong foundation of health and clarity, your intuition prospers.

Lesson 37

Haven

Activate your safe place.

Everyone desires a place to sleep that is safe and comfortable. Your bedroom is your haven, a place to relax and rejuvenate, a special place that is personal, private, and above all else, necessary. If you sleep 8 hours, you spend one third of your time in your bedroom. The exercise today is to evaluate your bedroom and how it provides rest.

Exercise 37-1: Bedroom

First, consider these areas of your bedroom:

1. *Bed.* Think not only of the mattress, its firmness/softness and size, but also of the location of the bed. Does it allow for movement in the room? Notice that the bed provides support for the whole body.

2. *Pillow.* Think of its softness and comfort. Maybe you have a non-allergenic or other special pillow. Notice that the pillow cuddles your head.

3. *Bedding.* Think of your blankets and sheets. Perhaps you use different sets at various times of the year. Notice that you select what is most comfortable and cozy.

4. *Temperature.* Think of heat and coolness. Notice that you like the temperature to be just right.

5. *Air.* Think of the freshness of the air. Notice whether you open windows, have plants, or run an air purifier.

6. *Light.* Think of the light in the room from windows, overhead lights, and lamps. Notice how you illuminate your bedroom.

7. *Darkness.* Think of how dark the room is. Notice how you shut out light.

8. *Sound.* Think of the sounds in the room, such as from a radio or from outside. Notice how you control the volume so you can sleep well and easily.

Second, evaluate your bedroom for ways to improve it if it doesn't feel as restful as you would like. Perhaps there is something from the list above such as a new pillow that you would like to change. Perhaps you can improve your comfort by removing some clutter. You can refresh your bedroom by changing just one thing. There is no need to tackle everything at once.

Exercise 37-2: Sleep

First, consider what you do before sleep:

1. *Finish activities.* Think of how you conclude your day. Perhaps you preview the next day's schedule. Or maybe you make lunches or plan tomorrow's meals.

2. *Prepare the house.* Notice how you ready your house for the night. Maybe you close all windows for quiet or open them for ventilation. You probably lock the doors so you are safe and turn out lights so it is dark.

3. *Transition time.* Think of what you do before getting into your bed. You remove shoes, jewelry, and glasses. Maybe you bathe, shower, and/or brush your teeth. You change into comfortable sleeping attire that doesn't restrict your body.

4. *Bedtime*. Be aware of what you do as you lie down. You slip between the sheets, pull up the bedding, put your head on your pillow, and close your eyes.

Second, evaluate your pre-bedtime habits for ways to improve them, if needed. One habit that helps tremendously is to eat your last meal two to three hours before going to sleep so you have time to digest your food. Then, notice how you sleep.

Summary

You take care of yourself by setting up your bedroom so that it is a place of repose—a haven. Every day you return to bed, an automatic process that allows your body to rest. Intuition doesn't get more basic than that—automatic, daily, and something that nurtures you.

Lesson 38

Opposites

We live in a world of opposites.

We make choices every day. Often we choose the opposite of what we are experiencing. When we overwork, we want to rest. We desire warm beverages on cold days and cold beverages on hot days. We put a cold pack on an injury to reduce inflammation. When our thinking is scattered, we try to gather our thoughts. If we have been sedentary too long, we get up and move.

Our study of opposites begins with the realization that they define each other, balance each other, and work with each other. When we increase our understanding of how opposites manifest in our lives, we understand how to better care for ourselves. We can more easily determine an appropriate diet, raise our consciousness, and enhance our intuitive ability.

Exercise 38-1: Observe Opposites

Notice how opposites appear in your daily activities. Pay attention to opposites; analyze how differences complement each other; determine how you react to things. Observe without judgment; no one quality is good or bad. Here are phenomena to consider; this list is by no means exhaustive:

◊ *Physical characteristics*: tall/short; fat/slender; hydrated/dehydrated.

◊ *Direction of growth*: up/down; vertical/horizontal.

◊ *Plant parts*: roots/stalk; leaves/flowers.

◊ *Emotional states*: laughing/crying; shy/expressive; agitated/calm; lethargic/energetic.

◊ *Mental states*: active learning/passive learning; eager/reticent.

◊ *Social activity*: extrovert/introvert.

◊ *Spiritual expression*: outward types with rituals/inner types with meditations.

◊ *Muscles*: contracting/expanding; biceps/triceps; quads/hamstrings.

◊ *Yoga exercises*: stretch one way/stretch the other way.

◊ *Cooking and diet choices*: warmth in cold times/cool in hot times; moisture in dry places/crisp and crunchy in moist places.

Exercise 38-2: Observe Spectrums

Recognize that opposites are endpoints of a range. For example, a rainbow has red at one extreme, violet at the other, and the whole spectrum of colors in between.

Here are some food categories and their respective spectrums.

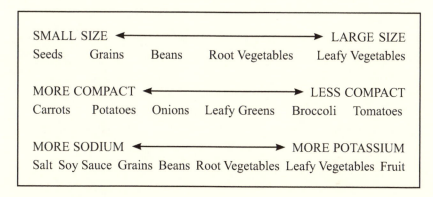

SMALL SIZE ◄————————————————► LARGE SIZE
Seeds   Grains   Beans   Root Vegetables   Leafy Vegetables

MORE COMPACT ◄————————————► LESS COMPACT
Carrots   Potatoes   Onions   Leafy Greens   Broccoli   Tomatoes

MORE SODIUM ◄————————————► MORE POTASSIUM
Salt Soy Sauce Grains Beans Root Vegetables Leafy Vegetables Fruit

Now, organize this list of legumes in a range from small to large size:
   ◊ azuki
   ◊ black-eyed pea
   ◊ fava
   ◊ garbanzo
   ◊ kidney
   ◊ lentil
   ◊ lima
   ◊ pinto
   ◊ soybean

Exercise 38-3: Observe Menu

Observe opposites in one of your meals today. Don't worry about labeling every item—merely look for some opposites. Consider a variety of foods and preparation methods, such as different categories of vegetables or cooking techniques.

Here are some examples:

   ◊ *Moisture content*: bread (hard and dry) versus soup (soft and moist).
   ◊ *Cooking method*: boiled rice (water cooking) versus stir-fried vegetables (oil cooking).

◊ *Textures*: pasta (al dente) versus sauce (smooth and creamy)

Summary

We live in a dualistic world of opposites. The study of opposites can heighten our intuition by increasing our understanding of the ranges of phenomena.

Note: Macrobiotic literature contains much useful information on opposites through the study of yin and yang. See *Essential Ohsawa* by George Ohsawa or *Essential Guide to Macrobiotics* by Carl Ferré for further study.

Lesson 39

Balance

Everything is important; yet nothing more so than anything else.

Career and family. Rest and exercise. Relationships and solo time. Balance occurs in life in our various responsibilities, desires, and activities.

Balance is a whole-life experience and is necessary for accomplishing what you want. The following exercise is repeated in lessons 40 and 41. For today, use the exercise to concentrate on your accomplishments and how you achieve balance in your life.

Exercise 39-1: What I Do Right—Accomplishments

Consider the following areas in your life to gain insight into how you maintain balance in your life by engaging in a variety of activities. You may find recalling examples easier in some areas than others, or that some areas are more positive than others:

Diet. Everyone needs to eat. Name one food that nourishes you.

Living quarters. Everyone needs a place to live, sleep, and keep belongings. Name something you really like about your house or living quarters.

People you live with. Everyone lives with others at some time. Think of a positive thing about one person you live with currently, or lived with in the past.

Physical exercise. Everyone needs movement. Name one physical activity that you enjoy.

Creativity. Everyone needs to feel they have contributed something—a project, writing, artwork, music, spontaneous doodling, etc. Name something you do to satisfy your creative needs.

Social needs. Everyone needs others, whether people or pets. Think of someone you socialize with.

Career. Everyone needs a job at one time or another. A job is a function, a place to work, a place of responsibility, and a place of fulfillment. Name something that is satisfying in the various jobs you do, or have done.

Education. Everyone is a product of learning. Think about your education—formal or otherwise—and name one thing that stimulates your mental capabilities.

Relaxation. Everyone needs downtime. Name something you do to relax.

Spiritual Fulfillment. Everyone needs enrichment. Consider your beliefs and name a practice such as meditation, an association such as a place of worship, or simply a philosophy that enriches you.

Play. Everyone needs time to play. Name something you do for fun or that makes you laugh.

Aesthetics. Everyone needs exposure to beauty, whether it be art, music, nature, or something else that generates appreciation, inspiration, creativity, or other wonders. Name one thing that lifts you up in this way.

Exercise 39-2: Analyze Reaction

After contemplating your accomplishments in the previous exercise, consider how you now feel towards yourself. Ideally, you experienced positive self-reflection and realized that your activities help you take care of yourself. Pay attention to any insights.

This is my favorite exercise to do when I need a pep talk or when I feel a need to encourage someone else. Success lies in thinking of specific examples with tangible results (taking a friend to lunch) as opposed to simply a general trait (being nice).

Summary

Taking care of yourself involves a balance of activities and a balanced attitude. All things you do and feel affect your insights and your personal growth, which in turn influence your intuition.

Lesson 40

Gentleness

There is no reason to be hard on yourself.

The last exercise was to evaluate different aspects of your life and see how they provide balance to create a well-rounded person. Each individual is a sum of parts, a balancing act of qualities. Today, we review the same aspects from another perspective. This reflective exercise provides an opportunity to look deeper into the overall balance of how you take care of yourself.

Exercise 40-1: What I Want to Improve—Ideal World

This exercise asks you to contemplate your desires; it may stimulate varied responses. Notice whether any of the answers are similar to those in Exercise 39-1. Consider the following areas of your life and think of one example of something you would do differently if given the chance:

Diet. Everyone needs to eat. Think of what you eat and name one food or food habit you wish were different.

Living quarters. Everyone needs a place to live, sleep, and keep belongings. Think of your house or living quarters and name something you would change if possible.

People you live with. Everyone lives with others at some time. Think of one thing you wish were different about someone you live with now or lived with in the past.

Physical exercise. Everyone needs movement. Name one activity you would like to change, do differently, or start doing.

Creativity. Everyone needs to feel they have contributed something—a project, writing, artwork, music, spontaneous doodling, etc. Name something you would change in fulfilling your creative needs.

Social needs. Everyone needs others, whether people or pets. Think of something you would like to be different with people in your life.

Career. Everyone needs a job at one time or another. A job is a function, a place to work, a place of responsibility, and a place of fulfillment. Name something you would change in your work or various jobs you do.

Education. Everyone is a product of learning. Think of something you would like to be different in your education and level of satisfaction.

Relaxation. Everyone needs downtime. Think of something you would like to change about what you do to relax.

Spiritual Fulfillment. Everyone needs enrichment. Think of something you would like to be different in your spiritual practices.

Play. Everyone needs time to play. Name one thing you would change about what you do for fun or to make you laugh.

Aesthetics. Everyone needs exposure to beauty, whether it be art, music, nature, or something else that generates appreciation, inspiration, creativity, or other wonders. Think of something you would change about the things that lift you up.

Exercise 40-2: Analyze Reaction

Consider how you feel towards yourself after completing the above exercise. Notice whether you feel differently now towards yourself and your achievements or lack of them.

This exercise can be positive if it helps you clarify things in your life for improvement. Resist the temptation to turn it into a negative complaint session. Pay attention to any reactions, both positive and negative. Finish the exercise by remembering there is value in analyzing aspects of your life and your attitudes about these aspects.

I really value this exercise when I need to get organized. At certain times of the year, I consider various aspects of my life so I can revise habits or identify areas for improvement. This is often very inspirational. However, I never do the exercise when I'm tired as it can degenerate into an exhaustive to-do list.

Summary

The aspects of your life define you. Whether you are praising yourself for all the things you do right or contemplating ways to improve, remember always to be gentle with yourself. Value your achievements and value your desires. In valuing these, you are strengthening your intuition about how you take care of yourself.

Lesson 41

In the Moment

What do you want?

Daily life constantly provides opportunities for spontaneous decision-making—decisions made in the moment. While many of our responses are habitual, they all are related to an intuitive awareness about what is an appropriate course of action. When we repeatedly choose the same actions, we reinforce intuitive awareness about what is useful and what isn't. This awareness helps when we need to make decisions quickly or about parts of our lives that aren't habitual.

Exercise 41: What do I Want? *Wow* and *Whoa*

Consider the areas of your life. Notice your feelings and thoughts as you answer the following questions. You may have positive feelings and thoughts such as, "Wow! I'm doing great!" You may have less-than-positive feelings and thoughts such as, "Whoa! I'm not doing as well as I hoped. I need to improve." You may be in a range in between. For the exercise today, notice whether your response is more of a *wow*, a *whoa*, or a combination:

Diet. Everyone needs to eat. Is your diet nourishing you?

Living quarters. Everyone needs a place to live, sleep, and keep belongings. Are you thriving in your house?

People you live with. Everyone lives with others at some time. Are (or were) you comfortable with your housemates?

Physical exercise. Everyone needs movement. Are you getting the right amount and kind of exercise?

Creativity. Everyone needs to feel they have contributed something—a project, writing, artwork, music, spontaneous doodling, etc. Are you doing things that meet your creative needs?

Social needs. Everyone needs others whether people or pets. Are you satisfying your social needs?

Career. Everyone needs a job at one time or another. A job is a function, a place to work, a place of responsibility, and a place of fulfillment. Are you fulfilled by your work?

Education. Everyone is a product of learning. Are you stimulated and inspired by the things you are learning, thinking about, reading, or studying?

Relaxation. Everyone needs downtime. Are you getting the right kinds and amount of relaxation?

Spiritual fulfillment. Everyone needs enrichment. Are your spiritual activities satisfying?

Play. Everyone needs time to play and laugh. Are you getting the right amount and kinds of play?

Aesthetics. Everyone needs exposure to beauty, whether it be art, music, nature, or something else that generates appreciation, inspiration, creativity, or other wonders. Are you inspired?

"What do I want?" is my favorite question when I need to make a decision quickly. It helps me by reminding me to pay attention to my intuitive awareness.

Summary

You have many areas in your life. You can think about them from various viewpoints. In the three prior lessons and exercises, you successively considered the same areas. In the first lesson, you thought about the areas in terms of satisfaction. In the next lesson, you thought of improvement in the areas. In the third, you considered your immediate situation and noted your reaction. These exercises are a way to practice intuitive awareness about how best to care for yourself.

Lesson 42

REVIEW: **Harmony**

When you care for yourself, you manage the details of your life and demonstrate love for yourself. Accepting all parts of yourself generates a feeling of harmony.

Let's review the past five lessons of this unit, lessons devoted to the theme of how you take care of yourself. Today, we recap the lessons and tie them together to help you realize how taking care of yourself is a result of your self-love.

Lesson 37: Haven. Your bedroom is your place of comfort, rest, and a haven for rejuvenation.

Lesson 38: Opposites. Opposites define all phenomena; both sides are necessary.

Lessons 39: Balance. When you acknowledge the things you do right, you appreciate how well-balanced you are.

Lesson 40: Gentleness. When you notice what you want, you notice how to improve yourself—be gentle in the process.

Lesson 41: In the moment. When you ask yourself what is needed in the moment, you tap into intuition and determine the best way to proceed.

You can use this method of review in many circumstances. For example, if you need a pep talk on a hard day, you can review all the things you do right. If you need to get organized, you can write a list of things to do. If you are making a difficult decision, you can ask yourself the question "What do I want at this particular moment?"

A second benefit of doing these exercises is to help you value the range of your responses and to appreciate all of them. Ideally, this prepares you to reduce, even eliminate, any conflict you have about different points of view. Accept that sometimes you think one way and other times you think another way. All of your perceptions are valuable and personally true for you. All can help you gain insight into how to help yourself. All can lead you to a place of peace, a feeling of harmony—the absence of conflict.

Love doesn't mean always feeling only one way. Rather, it means accepting all feelings. When you feel harmony about the varied aspects in your life and your innumerable feelings, you take care of yourself in an important way. Complete acceptance demonstrates your unconditional love for yourself.

Intuition is a way to tap into your inner knowingness about how to care for yourself; it fosters more acceptance of, and unconditional love for, yourself.

Exercise 42: Experience Now

It is important to recognize that unconditional love is always available for everyone, at every moment. This exercise cultivates that recognition, and it takes only three to four minutes.

Take a breath of air and inhale deeply; let your belly expand as you inhale. Exhale and let your belly relax. Inhale again and appreciate the air. In your mind's eye, see the sky above you. Notice that the sky reaches to the horizon...in front of you, behind you, above, and on all sides—all around you. Acknowledge that the atmosphere reaches all the way around the earth. Our atmosphere provides the environment needed for human life to exist. No one is excluded: rich and poor, young and old, man and woman, slave and free, people at war and people at peace. Everyone lives on earth and has access to air to breathe.

Our atmosphere can be viewed as a symbol of unconditional love. With every breath, you partake of the same atmosphere as everyone else. Connect with the life force around the planet and appreciate the love that is here.

Summary

Accept that you have a range of emotions. Tap into your notion of what is appropriate for you and cultivate feelings of gentleness toward yourself. Take care of your needs. Understand you are strong and have intuition. Let your intuition help you be at peace about what happens in your life.

Appendix 1

◊ *Intuition about Shopping*

Throughout your life, you have purchased food. Consider what you buy and what you avoid. Your selections are based on a certain set of criteria formed from your intuition—what you believe to be of benefit and what you habitually do. This course elaborates on many ways to increase intuition. One way is to start paying attention to which foods increase vibrancy and help you thrive.

The foods in the chart on page 161 are recommended as the basis for a healthy diet. Use it as a starting point for your shopping and eating. Note that while this list is vegan and many of the foods require preparation, animal foods and products and ready-to-eat foods can be part of a healthy diet as discussed later. Later in the course, we will explore more about each food category.

Seasonal fruits and vegetables. Fruits and vegetables have better flavor and vibrancy when in season; think of a tomato fresh from the vine compared to a tomato purchased in the winter at the store. If you garden or buy from a farmers' market, the selection is necessarily seasonally based. If you rely on store-bought produce, follow this general guideline to purchase seasonal foods:

Spring: Lettuces, radishes, early onions, peas, cherries, apricots, strawberries.

Summer: Cucumbers, summer squashes, fresh corn, green beans, tomatoes, peaches.

Fruits	Vegetables	Grains	Beans
Apples	Avocado	Barley	Azuki beans
Bananas	Broccoli	Breads	Blackeyed peas
Berries	Cabbage	Brown rice	Black turtle beans
Citrus fruit	Carrot	Buckwheat	Chickpeas
Coconut	Cauliflower	Corn & products	Green peas
Dates	Celery	Millet	Lentils
Figs	Garlic	Oats	Navy beans
Grapes	Greens	Pastas	Pinto beans
Peaches	Lettuces	Quinoa	Soy beans & products:
Pears	Mushrooms	Whole wheat &	tofu & tempeh
Raisins	Onions	products	White beans
	Potatoes		
	Squashes		
	Tomatoes		

Seeds/Butters	Nuts/Butters	Oils	Packaged Goods
Pumpkin seeds	Almonds	Coconut oil	Breads
Sesame seeds	Cashews	Olive oil	Miso
Sunflower seeds	Peanuts	Sesame oil	Natural sweeteners
Tahini	Peanut butter		Pickles, condiments
	Pecans		Sea salt
	Walnuts		Soy sauce
			Spices

Autumn: Winter squashes, turnips, carrots, apples, pears.

Winter: Fruits and vegetables that keep such as roots, squashes, apples.

Many vegetables such as broccoli, kale, and green onions are shipped from warmer locales and are available in stores year round. Learn what is grown in your area and choose food accordingly. If there are times of the year when nothing grows, use vegetables such as roots, onions, and cabbage that store well.

Organic fruits and vegetables. Organic foods have no pesticide residue. While it is worthwhile to purchase organic, if it is not available or cost is prohibitive, do your best to avoid the worst offenders.

Buy organic. These items are notorious for pesticide residue		Okay to buy if not organic. These items have little pesticide residue or are peeled before use	
Apples	Peaches	Avocadoes	Cucumbers
Celery	Potatoes	Bananas	Garlic
Grapes	Strawberries	Broccoli	Onions

Dried beans, grains, nuts, and seeds. These foods form the basis for a healthy diet in this course. They provide complex carbohydrates, proteins, fats, and fiber. You may be familiar with grains such as brown rice and rolled oats (oatmeal), beans such as split peas and lentils, and nuts and seeds such as almonds and sunflower seeds. If cooking these foods is new for you, then start slowly and follow the exercises in this course.

Fresh breads. Everyone loves bread; the best is made from superior ingredients such as whole grain flours, sprouted grains, and natural leavenings. Inferior breads include refined flours, additives, preservatives, artificial ingredients, sugars, and trans-fats. Read labels carefully and avoid these ingredients.

Oils. Oils help in cooking to make food delicious. Buy quality oils— the best ones are organic and unrefined. The two aspects that define quality oils are the source of the oil and the manufacturing process. For the best source, choose organic and non-GMO products. For the best manufacturing, choose oils using the least number of techniques and the most mechanical, rather than chemical, processing.

Oils originate from the germ of nuts and/or seeds—the small part of the plant that stores nutrients and fats and which the plant uses to form a new sprout. Pesticide residue is condensed in the germ, which contains all the genetic information. Genetically modified organisms (GMOs) produce seeds that cannot reproduce—seeds that provide questionable oils. Most, if not all, commercial corn, canola, and soy oils are genetically modified. Some oils come from cotton and peanuts, which are grown with high amounts of pesticides.

Another important aspect for oil is how it is made. The simplest method is cold-pressing and then packaging. Extra virgin olive oil (EVOO) is the first pressing from olives. Unrefined sesame oil comes from pressing sesame seeds. Unrefined coconut oil is packaged without heating. Other quality oils include flax, hazelnut, avocado, and almond.

Most commercial oils undergo more manufacturing. They are refined to create a neutral flavor and a long shelf life. Some companies use hexane, a petroleum product, to separate oil from the seeds. This solvent is used in the manufacture of safflower, soy, peanut, and corn oils.

Use logic to determine what oils to use. Cost is one consideration. Bear in mind that commercial enterprises strive for maximum quantity at minimum expense. Not surprisingly, inexpensive oil is often an inferior product. Labeling is another consideration. Buy oils from reputable suppliers and look for the words "organic" and "cold-pressed" as well as the pressing date on the label. Especially, look for oils labeled "non-GMO." Packaging is yet another issue. Oils are very fragile because the molecules break down easily with high heat and light. Choose oils that are bottled in a can or dark glass, which protects against light. Last but not least, taste oil to determine whether or not you want to use it.

Animal and dairy foods. Let your intuition guide you in whether or not to consume animal and/or dairy foods. If you do, buy the best quality possible. All animal foods concentrate pesticide residue; many animals are fed GMO feeds. Farmed fish are notorious for containing pesticides. Buy organic animal foods and products from reputable sources—the more local the better.

Packaged goods. Packaged foods make food preparation easy. However, there is a wide variety of selections—some healthy, others unhealthy. Learn to pay close attention to what is written on packaged food labels. Here are two lists that identify some undesirable ingredients.

Avoid These Items	Limit These Items
Artificial flavors	Caffeinated drinks and teas
Artificial sweeteners	Fried foods
Flavor enhancers such as MSG	Natural sugar, dehydrated cane juice
Genetically modified organisms (GMOs)	Overly salty snacks
High fructose corn syrup	Refined flours
Hydrogenated oils and trans-fats	
Preservatives	
Refined sugar	

Reading labels. Here are general tips for specific items to notice when reading labels:

1. *Number of ingredients*. In general, the more ingredients listed, the more processed the food.

2. *Type of ingredients*. Foods with unrecognized or unpronounceable ingredients are less desirable.

3. *Order of ingredients*. Items are listed from greatest to least quantity. Choose foods that have the greatest percentage of quality ingredients.

4. *Marketing*. There may be discrepancies between what is featured on the front of the package and where that ingredi-

ent is listed. Notice the relative quantity of a special high-lighted ingredient.

5. *Nutritional data.* Check for salt, fat, and sugar. Most products have more of these three ingredients than you would use if you made it yourself.

6. *Serving size.* Consider the actual amount of the nutrients you consume based on the quantity you will actually eat.

7. *What isn't there.* This is the hardest item to determine from labels—what they don't say. Oil labels often don't reveal the manufacturing process; GMO information is usually lacking; animal foods don't indicate the kind of feed. If the label doesn't say, "100 percent whole wheat (oat, etc.) flour," then the bread contains refined flour. Recognize there is a constant need for more information and education.

8. *Do your best.* Sometimes it is important to be vigilant; other times it is enough to feed yourself without excessive worry. Apply these tips with the underlying goal of taking care of yourself.

Summary. Intuition helps you choose what to buy. It helps you define healthy food versus unhealthy food. It helps you make logical choices and pick vibrant foods. Healthy food is a long-term investment in your future. Intuition helps you navigate the journey.

Appendix 2

◊ *Basic Menus*

Following are examples of light, medium, and full menus that satisfy caloric needs. Different people need differing amounts of food on a regular basis as well as at different times of day and when engaging in different activities than usual. For example, one elderly friend prefers a medium size breakfast, large lunch, and small dinner. This pattern is a change from an earlier time in her life when she had a small breakfast, medium lunch, and large dinner. Athletes, pregnant women, and growing children have varying needs too. Let your needs determine how much you need to eat.

Breakfast	Light	Medium	Full
Option 1	Toast Peanut butter Jam Tea	Toast Scrambled tofu or eggs Tea	Miso soup, full bowl Brown rice Toast with spread Greens Tea
Option 2	Toast Greens	Oatmeal Nuts or seeds Raisins or other dried fruit	Fried rice with tofu and vegetables Greens

166

Lunch	Light	Medium	Full
Option 1	Vegetable soup Green salad	Vegetable soup Full sandwich	Bean or minestrone soup Full sandwich
Option 2	Green salad Crackers Hummus	Grain or pasta salad	Pasta Sauce Vegetables

Snack	Light	Medium	Full
Option 1	Fresh fruit	Dried fruit	Dried fruit and nuts

Dinner	Light	Medium	Full
Option 1	Lentil soup Corn bread Vegetables	Brown rice Beans Stir-fried vege- tables	Fish or chicken Pasta and vegetables Salad
Option 2	Pasta Vegetables	Bean soup Brown rice Salad	Any meal with dessert

◊ *Intuition about Cooking*

When you use intuition in the kitchen, cooking becomes even more enjoyable and rises to another level. "Intuitive cooking" means going with the flow of the moment. It doesn't mean excluding cookbooks, measurements, or timing, although cooking without them is a wonderful way to hone your intuitive skills.

When cooking from recipes, pay attention to details so you know how to repeat the desired end product. Become familiar with your stove and pans so that you can succeed when cooking a different amount, using a different pan, or cooking in a different environment. This paves the way for cooking without measurements and relying more on intuition as your guide. Intuition also helps when you alter or modify recipes

It is helpful to learn how to prepare basic foods such as grains, beans, nuts and seeds, and vegetables and fruits. This will help you establish a foundation from which to expand your skills. The pages that follow provide an introductory primer on these foods.

◊ *Intuition about Grains*

Source. Whole grains provide complex carbohydrates and complete protein when eaten with beans.

Shopping. Look for grains with good color and shape, preferably within one year of harvest. Organic grains are preferred because they have higher amounts of nutrients, no pesticide residue, and taste better.

Measuring. Different grains require different amounts of water in preparation. The proportion decreases when cooking four or more cups or when pressure cooking. The proportion increases when making porridge.

Timing. Grains must be cooked until tender; timing varies per grain. Generally, whole grains require more time than polished, cut, or rolled grains.

Grain	Water	Time	Yield
1 cup barley	4 cups	1 hour	4 cups
1 cup brown rice	2 cups	1 hour	3 cups
1 cup buckwheat	2 cups	30 minutes	3½ cups
1 cup couscous	1¼ to 1½ cups	5 minutes	3 cups
1 cup millet	3 cups	30 minutes	4 cups
1 cup oatmeal	2½ cups	15 minutes	2½ cups
1 cup polenta	3 cups	20 minutes	3¼ cups
1 cup quinoa	2 cups	20 minutes	4 cups
1 cup whole oats	3 to 4 cups water	1 hour	3 to 4 cups

Cooking

1. *Grain first.* Put grain in water and bring to a boil. Add a pinch of salt per cup of grain. Simmer in a covered pan over low heat for suggested time.

2. *Water first.* Bring water to a boil first. Then, add salt and then add grain. Simmer in covered pan over low heat for suggested time.

Intuitive Tips

1. These two methods provide different results and are suggested as an intuitive exercise later in this course.

2. Barley, brown rice, millet, quinoa, and whole oats taste better when washed and drained before cooking to remove dust.

3. Barley, brown rice, and whole oats cook and digest better when soaked first. The exercise in Lesson 27 elaborates on this idea.

4. Grains cook better when left undisturbed. Don't stir or lift lid while boiling.

5. Sea salt helps grain cook and taste better. Practice pinch-

ing salt. Grab some salt with your fingers then measure it so you know the quantity of your pinch. This gives you a standard so you can intuitively pinch salt and other seasonings.

6. Measure grain-to-water ratio intuitively with the "knuckle method." To do this, first use a measuring cup to measure grain then water and put in pot. Then, place finger in pot to determine height of water above the grain. Next time, just use your finger to measure. You can expand on this exercise by using a different pan and noticing if the same knuckle measurement applies.

7. Develop intuitive ability in kitchen by paying attention to different smells as grains cook. The steam coming off the pot has an aroma that changes from beginning to end.

8. The chart is a starting point for intuitive ability. Adjust proportions of water and time for your needs and purpose.

Other Recipes and Ideas

1. Cook porridge overnight in a crockpot for breakfast. Use ½ cup whole oats or brown rice to 5 cups water, a 1-to-10 proportion. Season with salt, cinnamon, and/or ginger.

2. Cook rice plain first thing in the morning while showering or exercising and use later in the day for rice salad or fried rice and vegetables.

3. *Couscous with vegetables*. Sauté vegetables of choice, add 1½ cups water and seasonings, boil 3 to 4 minutes until vegetables are tender. Add 1 cup couscous and remove from heat. Let sit 5 minutes covered before serving.

◊ *Intuition about Beans*

Source. Beans provide protein and some fat.

Shopping. Look for beans with good color and shape, without an overabundance of broken pieces. Avoid beans that are colored with dyes.

Measuring. Beans require enough time and water to cook thoroughly. Begin with measurements, and add water when cooking as necessary so beans are covered.

Seasoning. Do not add salt to beans until near the end of the cooking time; salt inhibits cooking.

Timing. Beans must be cooked until soft. Timing varies per bean. Generally, the larger the bean, the longer it takes.

Bean	Water	Time	Yield
1 cup azuki beans	3 cups	1 hour	3 cups
1 cup black turtle beans	3 cups	1½ hours	2½ cups
1 cup chickpeas	3 cups	1½ hours	3 cups
1 cup lentils	3 cups	1 hour	2½ cups
1 cup pinto beans	3 cups	1½ hours	2½ cups
1 cup split peas	3 cups	1 hour	2½ cups

Cooking

1. *Boiling beans*. Bring beans and water to a boil. Simmer in pan with cover ajar to prevent overflow. Simmer for time specified or until completely soft. Add water as needed to

cover beans during cooking. Add sea salt and other seasonings only after beans are soft.

2. *Crockpot Cooking.* Use a crockpot to cook beans all day;
   when soft, add seasonings.

Intuitive Tips

1. Beans taste better when washed and drained first.

2. Whole beans cook and digest better when soaked first.
   Soaking removes phytic acid and improves digestibility.
   Soak 4 to 8 hours, then discard the soaking water and use
   fresh water.

3. Kombu sea vegetable helps soften beans as they cook, especially azuki, black turtle, chickpeas, and pinto. Kombu
   adds beneficial minerals and blends with the flavor of
   beans. This helps remove gas.

4. Beans must be soft before adding sea salt. Salt prevents
   beans from softening if used too early.

5. Grains and beans served in the same meal provide complete protein. This is important for growing children, pregnant women, and most people who are physically active.

Other Recipes and Ideas

1. *Pea soup.* Cook peas until soft. Add vegetables, seasonings, and sea salt.

2. *Pinto beans.* Soak beans. Cook until soft. Add seasonings
   and sea salt.

3. Explore using various herbs and spices when cooking
   beans. This is a great way to practice intuitive skills.

4. Practice cooking soup with beans and/or leftover broth
   and other ingredients. Cooking soup is a wonderful way to
   practice intuitive cooking.

◊ *Intuition about Nuts and Seeds*

Source. Nuts and seeds provide quality fats.

Shopping. Buy organic nuts and seeds with good color and shape within one year of harvest; they tend to become rancid with age. If buying whole nuts, look for consistent shape without an overabundance of broken pieces.

Measuring. Nuts and seeds have a higher proportion of fat than grains and beans. Use a small amount for garnish or in dishes.

Timing. Preparation time varies. For roasting nuts and seeds, generally the smaller the seed or nut, the less time required.

Cooking

1. *Roast on top of stove*. Place one kind of a nut or seed in dry skillet over medium heat. Stir constantly until roasted to preference, from 5 to 10 minutes.

2. *Roast in oven*. Place one layer of any kind of nut or seed on a baking sheet. Roast at 350 degrees for 7 minutes or longer, stirring occasionally.

3. *Nut milk*. Use 1 cup almond or cashews per 4 cups water. Pulse in blender and strain.

Intuitive Tips

1. Soaking removes phytic acid from nuts and improves digestibility. Soak 4 to 8 hours, then discard soaking water. Roast nuts as above or make nut milk with fresh water.

2. To save time and energy, roast seeds or nuts when oven is

already on and you're baking something else. Save for later use.

Other Recipes and Ideas
1. *Roast nuts and seeds.* Walnuts, sunflower seeds, almonds, or cashews. Roast and sprinkle with soy sauce.

2. *Dressings and dips.* Soak cashews or sunflower seeds. Pulse with garlic, green onion, and umeboshi or soy sauce, and other herbs and spices. Add water as needed for desired consistency.

◊ *Intuition about Vegetables and Fruits*

Source. Fruits and vegetables provide vitamins, minerals, color, fiber, refreshment, and flavor and are alkaline forming.

Shopping. Use common sense (intuition) about what you will realistically eat. Buy fruits and vegetables in season and choose vibrant items that appeal to you.

Measuring. Use common sense (intuition) about the quantity to prepare. It is easiest to use complete units such as 1 apple, 6 mushrooms, 1 basket of berries, 1 stalk of broccoli, or 1 handful of green beans. Notice how much you eat so that you can estimate how much to prepare when cooking for guests.

Timing. For optimal vitamins and minerals, serve both cooked and raw foods. Raw foods offer vitamins and minerals as nature intended; many fruits are best eaten raw, as are vegetables used in salads. Cooking is necessary for some vegetables to help make vitamins and minerals available. Cooking softens the fiber walls so digestion is easier. While overcooking is not recommended for vegetables such as broccoli, thorough cooking is preferred for vegetables such as winter squash or sweet potatoes and can enhance sweetness, palatability, and culinary use. When timing the cooking of vegetables, note that different vegetables, modes of preparation, quantities, and size of pieces affect the timing. These variations are wonderful ways to sharpen intuitive skills.

Cooking

1. *Steam vegetables*. Place ½ inch water in pan. Insert steamer basket and vegetables. Steam to desired tenderness.

2. *Stir-fry vegetables*. Heat oil and sauté vegetables, stirring often. Add one vegetable at a time, starting with the most dense. Cook until tender; add water and cover pan if desired. Season with soy sauce at end.

3. *Simmer vegetables*. Boil ½ inch of water in pan. Add vegetables and simmer until tender. Corn, green beans, carrots, and sweet potatoes are wonderful this way.

4. *Blanch vegetables*. Boil 2 cups of water in pan. Immerse vegetables in water and bring to a boil, simmer briefly. Blanched greens are superb.

5. *Bake vegetables*. Cut vegetables into bigger pieces or French fry shapes. Coat with a small amount of oil. Bake at 350 degrees until tender.

6. *Raw vegetables*. Combine lettuce with other fresh young vegetables for fresh salads.

7. *Fruit salads*. Choose 2 or more kinds of fresh fruit and cut into bite-sized pieces. Sprinkle fresh lemon or orange juice on top if needed to retain color.

8. *Fruit sauces*. Cut fresh fruit such as apples, pears, and ber-

ries, add a little water, and simmer until soft with salt, cinnamon, and vanilla or other seasonings. Purée if desired.

9. *Stewed compotes.* Simmer in a little water dried fruit such as apricots, plums, peaches, or cherries with seasonings such as ginger, coriander, or lemon zest until soft.

10. *Dried fruit and nuts.* Combine favorite kinds for a snack—almonds and dates, walnuts and raisins, cashews and cherries, or other combinations of choice.

Intuitive Tips

1. Match cooking style with personal preference. Do you like steamed vegetables? Stir-fried? Baked?

2. Wash vegetables in a basin of water rather than under a running faucet. Greens, spinach, and lettuce clean more thoroughly this way.

3. Learn to use a vegetable knife and to cut vegetables in more than one way.

4. Time cooking without a clock.

5. Make good use of your time. This is obvious, but many people omit fresh vegetables because they feel they take too much time. Prepare vegetables by washing and cutting into bite-sized pieces when you return from shopping. Use within a day or two. Prepare extra vegetables at dinner and eat for lunch the next day. Prepare a stewed compote or sauce and use for dessers or snacks over a few days.

Appendix 3

◊ *Intuition about Salt and Spices*

Source. Salt, herbs, and spices provide not only flavor but, in small amounts, they also improve the health-giving properties of your food. For example, salt facilitates cooking of grains and adds an alkaline factor to beans. Salt is absent in most home-cooked foods unless added. In ready-to-eat food, it is often present in excessive quantities. Herbs and spices add fragrance and flavor, stimulate digestion, and can aid digestion.

Shopping. Buy the best quality sea salt, herbs, and spices that you can find because they can vary in quality. The best sea salts, such as Celtic grey, retain trace minerals. Herbs and spices are best when fresh or freshly dried. When you open a jar of dried herb or spice, the fragrance should waft out. Green leafy herbs lose freshness faster than more spicy ones like pepper and cinnamon. However, even pepper and cinnamon lose pungency after time. Replace dried herbs and spices when the fragrance is gone. By buying from bulk bins in a natural foods store, you can buy small quantities at low prices.

Measuring. It is wonderful to employ your intuition when using sea salt, herbs, and spices. Recipes may prescribe quantities but you can learn to gauge the correct amount to suit your taste and preference. Too much or too little make a difference. One way to measure is grasp an amount between thumb and forefinger, i.e., "pinch measure." Use a big or little pinch according to what seems appropriate to you.

Another way to use herbs and spices is to smell the food as it cooks.
Hold an herb or spice (one at a time) above the pot and compare the
smell of the cooking food with the aroma of the spice. If they smell
compatible, add a small pinch at a time until it feels right.

Timing. Some seasonings are best added at the beginning, especially
for deep flavor: think ginger, cumin, and garlic. Add others at the
end: consider dried dill or fresh herbs. Other seasonings are used
without cooking, such as fresh garlic in hummus. Sea salt is better
when added as the food cooks rather than sprinkled on later at the
table. Use the proper amount to flavor the food.

Intuitive Tips
1. Take the sea salt test. Let your intuition guide you in which
   sea salt to use. Sample a few grains and analyze for flavor
   and reaction. Sea salt should taste wonderful and not harsh.
   If you test more than one kind in succession, sip water between tasting.

2. Take the herb and spice test. Let your intuition guide you in
   which ones to use. For dried products, smell the fragrance,
   which should be full, and select ones that appeal to you.
   For fresh products, look for vibrancy and aroma. Organic
   herbs and spices are free from pesticides and fillers.

General Recipes to Practice Intuitive Skills
1. *Gomashio*. This condiment is made with roasted sesame
   seeds and sea salt. It is delicious over cooked grains, pastas,
   and vegetables. To prepare: Dry-roast ½ cup whole brown
   or black unhulled sesame seeds in a skillet without oil. Stir
   constantly until the seeds are popping and fragrant, about 5
   to 7 minutes. Place in a blender with 1 to 2 teaspoons of sea
   salt and pulse to a coarse powder. If sea salt is moist, dry
   roast in skillet and/or pulse in blender first.

2. *Pesto*. This topping for pasta is traditionally made with

garlic, roasted pine nuts, fresh basil, olive oil, salt, and Parmesan cheese, but lends itself well to substitutions and adaptations. Try fresh cilantro instead of basil; add fresh parsley; use roasted walnuts or almonds in place of pine nuts; use miso or umeboshi in place of salt and Parmesan cheese. Proportions can vary to provide satisfying results. Recipe: ½ cup nuts, 4 cups basil, 6 tablespoons olive oil, 2 tablespoons miso, and crushed garlic.

3. *Salad dressing.* Make your own signature salad dressings with olive oil, vinegar, and herbs and spices. Use 3 parts oil to 1 part vinegar; add herbs and spices of your choice.

4. *Stir-fry vegetables with spices.* Start with finely chopped fresh ginger, whole cumin seeds, and/or curry powder in oil; then add vegetables. Be sure the spices don't burn. Season with soy sauce at end.

◊ *Intuition about Oils*

Source. Oils provide fats and help foods taste delicious.

Shopping. Oils vary by source and production. The following table lists commonly available oils and their source of production. Mechanical extraction, labeled as expeller-pressed and/or cold-pressed on packaging, involves pressing and crushing, either with rollers or a screw-type press. Mechanical pressing can generate heat due to friction, but no extra heat is used. It is the preferred method of extraction. Solvent extraction involves the use of hexane or other chemicals to separate the oil. After extraction, the solvent is removed, although it is questionable how much residue remains.

After extraction, either mechanical or solvent, oils can be further refined. If so, they are heated to a high temperature, deodorized, and sometimes bleached.

Shop for the highest quality oils you can find. Choose organic oils because commercial and non-organic oils contain pesticide residue. Also select oils labeled "Expeller Pressed" or "Cold Pressed." Insist on unrefined oils because oils are heated when refined, often to the point of denaturing.

Oil	Type of fatty acid	Production	Notes	Uses
Coconut oil	Saturated	Mechanical	First pressing is called extra virgin.	Baking and frying; stable oil.
Corn oil	Polyunsaturated	Mechanical or solvent	Corn is often genetically modified.	Oil is usually refined. Not recommended.
Cottonseed oil	Polyunsaturated	Solvent	Cotton is usually grown with pesticides.	Not recommended.
Olive oil	Monounsaturated	Mechanical	First pressing is called extra virgin.	All-purpose; light cooking and dressings.
Palm oil	Saturated	Mechanical	Often is refined after pressing.	Hard to find for home use; used in products.
Palm kernel oil	Saturated	Mechanical and solvent	Byproduct of palm oil production.	Hard to find for home use; used in confections.
Peanut oil	Monounsaturated	Mechanical followed by solvent	Comes from peanuts not good enough to be ground into peanut butter.	Used in high-heat cooking in restaurants; not recommended.
Rapeseed (canola)	Polyunsaturated	Mechanical or solvent	Seeds are genetically modified.	Not recommended.

Oil	Type of fatty acid	Production	Notes	Uses
Safflower oil	Polyun-saturated	Mechanical or solvent	High oleic variet-ies were develop-ed by selective hybridizing.	Often refined. Used in high-heat cooking, but hard to find unrefined
Soybean oil	Polyun-saturated	Solvent	Soybeans are genetically modi-fied.	Oil is usually refined. Used by most restaurants; not recommended
Sunflower oil	Polyun-saturated	Mechanical	High oleic variet-ies were devel-oped by selective hybridizing.	High-heat cook-ing for occasion-al use.
Gourmet oils: almond, avocado, walnut, etc.	Polyun-saturated	Mechanical	Specialty oils.	Use without heating.
Grapeseed oil	Polyun-saturated	Mechanical and solvent	By-product of wine industry.	Pesticide residue; use with dis-cretion.
Rice bran oil	Monoun-saturated and polyunsatu-rated	Mechanical	Comes from rice.	Hard to find.
Supplement oils: flax, herbs	Polyun-saturated	Mechanical	Fragile oils that denature easily with any heat.	Buy in black container. Re-frigerate.

Measuring. It is wonderful to use intuitive measurements (eyeballing the amount) for salad dressings, sautéing, and baking. Proportions are important for baked goods but, with practice, you can intuitively measure those amounts too.

Timing. Use care in cooking with liquid oils. Heat higher than 212 degrees F. denatures (damages) the oil, so sauté for short times and at medium- to-low heat. When baking, use cocnut oil as it can withstand higher temperatures.

Intuitive Tips

1. Take the taste test. The easiest and most accurate way to determine whether a specific oil is appropriate for you is to sample a small amount. Taste oil to determine whether it has a delicious flavor and smooth feel in swallowing. If oil tastes rancid, it is old and should be discarded. If oil has a chemical flavor or feel, it was processed with solvents.

2. Use care when frying. If oil gets too hot, it can spit, smoke, and become toxic. If this happens, remove pan from heat and discard oil. Wipe pan clean. Begin again.

General Recipes to Practice Intuitive Skills

1. *Salad dressing*. Make your own salad dressings with oil and vinegar. Experiment with different oils and vinegars and herbs and spices. Use 3 to 4 parts oil to 1 part vinegar.

2. *Fried rice*. Sauté fresh garlic, ginger, and mushrooms until done, add soy sauce, then leftover cooked rice with green scallions and heat through.

3. *Cookies*. If you have a favorite cookie recipe, try preparing it without measuring, eyeballing the proportions and intuit-ing the consistency of the dough.

◊ *Cravings*

In a course on intuition, it is important to discuss internal signals or urges. Generally, we interpret internal signals as positive or negative—a positive urge is labeled "intuitive" and a negative one "craving." All internal urges are signals that the body needs something. In an ideal world, a person would eat according to positive drives (intuition) and receive all nutrition and satisfaction. Negative drives (cravings) wouldn't even arise. This is one of the goals of this course—to help you identify your internal needs in order to satisfy and create a healthy body. A healthy body helps your spiritual self flourish and grow; in turn, your spiritual self helps your body. This is a wonderful cycle between body and soul, where positive urges (intuition) are the connecting thought.

Cravings are urges that drive us to eat undesirable foods, unhealthy items, or abnormal quantities. Because cravings can cause uncontrollable behavior, they can lead to guilt, frustration, low self-esteem, and unhealthy consequences, especially when we consume something very unhealthy or a large quantity. Definitely, these are the types of cravings to change. Even so, these types of cravings are signals that the body is in need.

Cravings, like intuition, are inner signals and should not be ignored; they can help us learn how to help ourselves. Start by noticing which cravings, if any, are problematic, i.e., cause you to go out of your way or forego bedtime or dominate your thinking until the craving is satisfied. It is easy to identify these cravings because they are so strong. Usually, simple "willpower" is not enough to overcome this level of craving because it signals a deeper need. By replacing negative urges with positive attitudes, behaviors, and foods, you use your intuition to help yourself.

There are cravings for many different foods, and they arise in different ways. I like to place them into three general categories:

One: Cravings of Timing

These cravings happen because of the time of life or because of bad timing on a particular day. Time of life cravings happen to people in certain ages and/or situations. Pregnant women crave certain foods because of changing needs caused by the growing baby. Children and teenagers also grow rapidly and crave certain foods. Women in their monthly cycles can have cravings related to hormonal swings. The best way to deal with these cravings is to be proactive in getting enough calories and nutrition so these cravings don't start or are minor and easy to deal with.

Cravings due to bad timing happen when a person misses a meal, accidentally or by choice, and the body responds by demanding food. This situation can happen after a fast, when sick, after skipping breakfast, or even after eating too little at the prior meal. Being without food can lead to low blood sugar and nutritional imbalances if frequent. The best way to deal with these cravings is to consume enough and the right kinds of calories. Seek a good meal immediately, such as whole-grain sandwich and soup. Be proactive in the future so it doesn't repeat.

Two: Nutritional Imbalances or Needs

Many cravings arise due to poor nutritional choices; there are many situations. Some situations are immediate—a person eats a big salad for lunch and then craves pastries afterwards. One situation happened to me all the time before I became aware: I'd eat a meal of rice, beans, and vegetables with no oil, nuts, or animal foods— a low-fat vegetarian macrobiotic feast. Afterwards, I would crave cookies and sweets. The best way to deal with these imbalances is to consume a small amount of the craved food in a healthy way—in this case, a healthy cookie. Be proactive in the future and eat well-balanced meals with adequate nutrition of complex carbohydrate, quality protein, and healthy fats.

When nutritional cravings are not met and imbalances happen over years, deficiencies can occur. People who eat animal foods without adequate whole grains and vegetables suffer health problems as do vegetarians without enough vitamin B_{12}. Children suffer on low-fat diets; people on strict diets sometimes go on binges of excessive sweets and/or alcohol.

Nutritional imbalances can produce other long-term effects. Here are some examples of long-term nutritional imbalances or cravings: Children raised in vegetarian households who begin eating a lot of red meat as adults. Children raised in households with a lot of meat who begin eating mostly raw foods as adults. Strict vegetarians who eat many sugary desserts. Many trendy diets are caused by long-term nutritional imbalances—for example, American diet to vegetarian to high meat consumption to raw foods to gluten-free. Often, the more dramatic the change, the more likely an underlying nutritional imbalance exists.

The best method for maintaining health is to eat carbohydrates, proteins, and fats in adequate quantities on a regular basis. This strengthens your intuitive ability to trust the feedback you receive. Cravings that once arose due to nutritional imbalances eventually even out.

Three: Absence and Desire—Addiction, Allergy, Detox, Elimination, Emotional

All of these types of cravings happen when your body is denied something it is accustomed to getting. The serious cravings come from addiction; without the food there is a reaction such as body spasms, uncontrollable behavior, and unreasonable emotions. The mind can't concentrate beyond the urge. Cravings for coffee, chocolate, alcohol, refined sugar, and some food additives vary from mild to extreme. The best way to deal with them is through willpower and intervention for serious cravings. More information follows in the section on "Addictions" in this appendix.

In allergy cravings, the body ironically desires the substance it reacts to, such as milk, chocolate, or oranges. In detox and elimination cravings, the body desires the food that is being purged. Prolonged fasts and cleanses can initiate these cravings. Emotional cravings are for comfort food. For emotional cravings, it is important to address the situation through means other than food, such as getting together with friends.

The charts of specific cravings on the following pages explain what the cravings mean and what to do about them.

MEAT **What craving means**	**What to do**
Need for protein, immediately.	Eat good quality meat within a nutritionally balanced meal of vegetables and grains. Or, eat higher proportion of beans within a nutritionally balanced meal of grains and vegetables.
Detox or elimination craving, especially if stopping animal foods.	Substitute flavors. Fried tempeh or seitan or portobello mushroom can be similar in taste and texture.
Need for protein, long term; if craving has gone on for years, there is an overall nutritional imbalance.	Need to increase protein quantity and quality overall.

DAIRY FOODS **What craving means**	**What to do**
Need for fat, immediately.	Eat small amount of quality fat of choice, such as organic cheese, yogurt, or milk within a nutritionally balanced meal. Or, get fat from vegetable sources such as olive oil, flaxseed oil, nuts, or seeds.
Allergic craving	Avoid all dairy foods. Use tofu in any way.
Detox or elimination craving, especially if stopping dairy foods.	To speed detox process, consume plenty of salad with olive oil and lemon juice.
Emotional craving for comfort food.	Substitute foods: For ice cream texture, make pudding. For ice cream coolness, make jelled desserts. For pizza and sandwiches, use imitation cheeses. In quiche, lasagna, and casseroles, use tofu. For beverages, use almond or rice milk.
Need for fat, long term. If craving has gone on for years, there is an overall nutritional imbalance.	Need to increase fat overall. Consume more high quality fat, such as olive oil dressings for vegetables, ghee for bread, nut butters in sauces, and nuts and seeds in snacks.
Need for calories especially for growing children, teenagers, athletes, and pregnant women.	Eat sufficient quantity of healthy foods with emphasis on quality fats and proteins.

COOKIES AND PASTRIES **What craving means**	**What to do**
Need for glucose, immediately. Low blood sugar from skipped meal.	Eat something quick and easy to digest, such as banana, juice, or dried fruit. Or, eat small amount of craved item. Or, fruit and nuts, peanut-butter-and-jelly. For long term, be proactive and don't skip meals. Eat whole grains for long-term steady source of carbohydrate.
Need for fat and protein, especially if craving occurs after full meal.	Eat small dessert. Or, eat dried fruit and nuts. Be proactive for long term and eat enough quality fat and protein in meals.
Need for sweet flavor.	Use more salt in cooking to bring out flavors, especially for whole grains.
Need for carbohydrate, immediately, especially after a meal with only salad.	Eat crackers and peanut butter. Be proactive in future and eat some protein and carbohydrate with salad.
Addictive craving, especially if craving is for particular cookie or pastry.	Identify addiction and wean. Or, substitute product.
Emotional craving for comfort.	Identify seriousness of craving. Address with comfort in other areas of life.
Need for calories.	Eat enough quality carbohydrates, fats, and proteins. Then eat healthy baked goods.

JUNK FOOD AND CANDY **What craving means**	**What to do**
Addicted to refined sugar, refined oils, caffeine, food additives, colorings, MSG, or other preservatives or chemicals.	Wean from products.
Need for glucose, immediately. Low blood sugar.	Substitute fruit or juice. Be proactive for future and eat regular meals and snacks of good quality.
Need for fat if craving is for high-fat junk food.	Substitute snack of better quality. Or, substitute dried fruit and nuts.

CHOLATE What craving means	What to do
CHOCOLATE **What craving means**	**What to do**
Addiction to caffeine and/or sugar.	Wean from products. Decrease how often eaten. Be proactive and consume a healthy diet over the long term.
Emotional craving for comfort.	Choose good quality chocolate over cheap chocolate. Eat a small amount and savor slowly.
Menstrual period (prior and during).	Eat a small amount and savor slowly. Be proactive and consume a healthy diet over the long term.
Possible need for magnesium.	Some people have suggested that chocolate cravings come from magnesium deficiency. Eat more leafy greens for magnesium.

COFFEE **What craving means**	**What to do**
Addiction to caffeine.	Wean slowly. Or, substitute with tea.
Addiction to cream, chocolate, or sugar in coffee.	Wean from the extra items.
Need for glucose. Low energy or blood sugar.	Sleep enough hours. Exercise daily. Eat healthy diet with enough flavor.

SPECIFIC FLAVORS AND TEXTURES **What craving means**	**What to do**
Sour flavor: Imbalance.	Wean from sour foods such as lemon, vinegar, pickles, which release calcium from bones. Eat more calcium-rich food and/or umeboshi.
Salty flavor: Addiction.	Use more salt and soy sauce in cooking. Wean from salted snacks.
Crunchy foods: Emotional need for comfort.	Substitute with healthy crunchy textures such as popcorn, nuts, and raw vegetables. Be proactive and consume regularly.

Do not fear your cravings or let them control you; they are merely signals that something needs to be taken care of. Pay attention to their strength. If they are mere whims, enjoy them. If they are bothersome and persistent, make corrections.

All inner signals, both positive intuitive ones and negative craving ones, are messages that can help you care for yourself. Do your best to instill good eating habits and consume quality foods; then negative cravings won't dominate your thinking or your life.

◊ *Addictions*

Addictions are cravings, or internal urges, that are more than inconveniences. They are harmful and potentially damaging. We commonly think of addictive behaviors as smoking, drinking alcohol, and overusing drugs. Eating foods that are detrimental to health is another form of addiction, even if not clinically or legally classified as such. White refined sugar, food additives, and caffeine in coffee, chocolate, and soda can create dependency, especially if consumed regularly for a period of time.

Addictions to these substances can interfere with intuition. They mask accurate interpretation of internal prompts because the addiction dominates choices. For example, when a person is addicted to caffeine, an internal thirst can prompt a person to seek coffee or soda rather than water. There are ways to deal with addictions. Here are general suggestions:

1. *Acknowledge addiction.* The first step is to admit there is an addiction. Signs of addiction include having to ingest the item regularly or else the body "demands" it. There may be physical symptoms of shaking or exhaustion, emotional outbursts or mood swings, or mental symptoms of denial or justification. If you ask other people whether they think you have an addiction and they agree, then take their perception seriously.

2. *Seek help.* The second step is to seek assistance, whether from doctor, therapist, internet, or self-help course. Some addictions require more intervention. While food addictions seem to be less serious than drug or alcohol addictions, they still create chaos and impede intuition. It is important to get information.

3. *Utilize willpower.* The third step, which is simultaneous with the second, is to acknowledge and use your own innate power. Everyone has inner strength to help them through hard times. Recognize you want to live and want to live well. Some addictions can be resolved through singular effort; others need a combined effort. Don't underestimate how powerful addictions are; but also, don't underestimate how much power you have.

4 and 5. *Purge the old and Establish the new.* The fourth and fifth steps are likewise simultaneous. Purge old patterns and establish new ones. How you implement the method is contingent on the seriousness of the addiction, your own willpower, and a reasonable timetable of accomplishment. See table on page 191.

6. *Spiritual connection.* Do addictions hide our spirituality or bring us closer? I've heard both views—that addiction masks the true nature, and that addictions create a high and this high is a way to connect with spiritual nature. Regardless of whether one or both are true, remember to be kind to yourself in the process of overcoming addiction. Recall also that 12 Step programs acknowledge a spiritual source for overcoming addictions. They stress reliance on a power greater than oneself for help.

Purge the old	Establish the new
Fast. Stop eating the food. Wean yourself from the addictive item, in stages if that is easier.*	Substitute. Eat new items that may be similar to old (if needed at first) for flavor, appeal, or other criteria. Learn, learn, learn.
Recognize triggers. Identify the situations and scenarios that stimulate addiction. Reduce exposure.	Incorporate healthy habits. Create rhythm and order to your schedule. Address nutrition. Exercise and drink enough water.
Program to detox. Set up a strategy for removing what you don't want and do what makes sense. Perhaps tackle the mild addictions first; maybe your health requires you to address the serious addictions first.	Program to change. Build levels of success within your program of change. Consider rewards and motivations that are worthwhile and reinforce healthy habits, such as a massage or movie with friends.

* There are many methods and techniques to rid oneself of food addiction. One way is through unpleasant association. For example, I associate fried doughnuts with the fat cellulite. Memories work well too. When I was a child, I had to take some awful tasting medicine, which made me gag. My mother tried to ease the taste with whipped cream, which I loved. I swallowed the medicine, then the cream, and then both came up. Now, I can't eat whipped cream without remembering the taste of that medicine.

Addiction, on some level, is an internal urge, a signal from your internal self of something you need. Let your urge come from a place of wholeness and health, a connection with the spiritual essence of life. In this way, let your intuition help you deal with and transform any addictions into knowledge and power to help you thrive.

Appendix 4

◊ *Glycemic Index*

The Glycemic Index ranks carbohydrates on a scale from 0 to 100 based on how much they raise blood sugar levels after eating. High GI foods are rapidly digested and absorbed; accordingly, they quickly and significantly increase glucose in the bloodstream, which is then followed by a rapid decline, i.e. the familiar "sugar high" and "sugar low." At the other end of the spectrum are low GI foods that are slowly digested and absorbed; accordingly, they gradually increase and gradually decrease glucose in the bloodstream. People with diabetes benefit from consuming a low GI diet because it stabilizes both glucose and lipid levels. Similarly, a low GI diet is beneficial for weight loss because the onset of hunger is gradual.

The GI is not a list of good carbohydrates and bad carbohydrates, where low numbers are preferred over high numbers. The GI merely indicates the quantity of glucose available in a food and the rapidity with which it will enter the blood. In addition, the GI doesn't present the entire nutrient profile of foods, although we can explain the data in reference to other nutrients. For example, beans generally have a lower GI ranking than whole grains. Both beans and grains have carbohydrate and protein. Beans have more moderate carbohydrate and higher protein than grains, which have higher carbohydrate and more moderate protein than beans.

Fiber also affects the GI. White rice has a slightly higher GI than brown rice. Orange and apple juice have higher numbers than oranges and apples. Vegetables have a range of carbohydrate; starchy vegetables such as sweet potato have more than green vegetables such as broccoli or lettuce. Generally, most fruits, vegetables, nuts, legumes, and whole grains are low GI; whole wheat products, basmati rice, and dried fruits are medium GI; and white breads and many boxed breakfast cereals are high GI.

Here is a sample of some foods on the Glycemic Index. Note: other sources may have slightly different numerical rankings. This chart includes comparisons of some foods.

Food	Glycemic Index	Comparisons
Brown rice White rice	66 to 87 83 to 93	Brown rice generally has a lower GI than white rice due to its fiber content. Specific kinds vary.
Rye bread White sourdough bread Whole wheat pita White bread	51 52 57 70	Breads vary depending on ingredients. Generally, the fewer the refined products, the lower the number.
Chickpeas Pinto beans	34 39	Beans have more protein than carbohydrate, thus a lower ranking.
Peanuts Cashews	14 22	Nuts have more fat and protein than carbohydrate, thus a lower ranking.
Sweet potato Baked russet potato	65 85	Potatoes vary considerably, depending on preparation and generally have more carbohydrate than other vegetables.
Corn tortilla Corn on cob Corn chips	52 53 72	Corn varies depending on product.
Grapes Raisins Apple Orange Apple juice Orange juice Banana, underripe Banana, overripe	46 64 38 42 40 50 30 52	Dried fruit condenses the carbohydrate. Juice has more carbohydrate than original fruit. The freshness of fruit affects the amount of carbohydrate.
Source: *Righthealth.com* and *Health.harvard.edu*		

◊ *Protein Needs for an Optimum Diet*

There are compelling reasons to be vegetarian and compelling reasons to eat animal foods. Here are a few ideas to consider:

1. *Teeth*. Adult humans have thirty-two teeth. Eight (¼) are incisors that cut into foods, perfect for fruits and vegetables. Four (⅛) are canine, which are pointed and useful for tearing into foods like meat. Twenty (⅝) are molars which are flat and useful for grinding. Some people cite the type and proportion of teeth as an indicator of an optimal diet: mostly grains, beans, and tubers followed by fruits and vegetables with minimal animal foods.

2. *Digestive tract*. A carnivorous animal such as a dog or cat has a digestive tract that is seven to nine feet long, ideal for assimilating and excreting meat in a short time. Humans have a longer tract, about twenty-eight feet long, which is suitable for longer digestion. Some people look to the example of length of digestive tract to indicate optimal diet—one based on plant foods and minimal, if any, animal foods.

3. *Traditional diets*. There are many traditional diets ranging from prehistoric cave dwellers to early civilizations to modern ethnic and cultural cuisines. Cavemen hunted animals and gathered roots, leaves, and fruits in season. Early civilizations tended crops of whole grain, fresh fruits, and vegetables, and raised their own animals. Modern ethnic cuisines favor regional foods.

   Traditional diets weren't vegan, but neither did they resemble modern-day patterns of animal food consumption. In traditional diets, animals were either wild or were raised in small numbers. In addition, animal foods were consumed as available, not necessarily for the majority of all meals. Seasonal crops were important. Foods weren't refined, especially for the masses, and never packaged, although items were dried and stored for later use.

Many long-lived cultures have been studied extensively, such as the Okinawans in Japan, or Russians in Soviet Georgia. A common pattern is consumption of local, mostly plant foods. While data is interpreted in various ways, the fact is that none of the diets is completely vegan—all include some animal foods, although not in major amounts and all with minimal processing.

Another pattern is seen with traditional cultures such as Hispanics or Japanese who immigrate to the United States and adopt a different diet. Hispanics originally ate rice, corn, beans, vegetables, and small amounts of meat. Upon coming to the U.S., they begin to eat poor quality animal foods, fast foods, processed foods, packaged goods, and sweets. Similarly, Japanese begin to eat more dairy foods and processed foods and eat less eating miso soup, rice, sea vegetables, and fish. In both populations, health suffers as obesity rises and diseases increase owing to the change to an inappropriate diet.

4. *Ethical reasons.* Some people avoid eating animals because animals suffer on factory farms. In modern times, this is a serious problem. High animal food consumption is linked to disease, overgrazing, and environmental pollution. Even though people have eaten animal foods since the beginning of time, the quality and circumstances around most animal foods has changed considerably.

5. *Authority.* Some inspirational teachers were vegetarian. Think of Thoreau or Gandhi. Some weren't, such as Martin Luther King, Jr. or Abraham Lincoln. Regardless of diet, it

is important to remember we can learn from everyone, and that both meat and no meat have their places.

◊ *Summary of Vitamins and Minerals*

Vitamins	Soluble in	Sources	Benefits	Notes
Vitamin A	Fat	Butter Egg yolks Liver Fish oils	Eyes Skin Tissues Antioxidant	Synthetic vitamin A is toxic in excess
Beta Carotene	Water	Carrots Winter squash Broccoli Leafy greens	Eyes Skin Tissues Antioxidant	Converts to vitamin A in the body
B Complex Thiamine (B_1) Riboflavin (B_2) Niacin (B_3) Pantothenic acid (B_5) Pyridoxine (B_6)	Water	Whole un-refined grains	Heart Nervous system Many digestive and metabolic processes	Usually found together
B_{12}	Water	Eggs Dairy products Meat Fish	Blood cells Nervous system	Vegans need to supplement
Folic Acid	Water	Leafy greens	Blood cell production	Important during pregnancy
Vitamin C	Water	Citrus fruits Bell peppers Cabbage Parsley Sprouts Other fruits and green leafy vegetables	Wound healing Common cold Tissue repair Capillary walls Powerful antioxidant	Heat destroys it Alcohol, drugs, and smoking reduce quantity in the body

Vitamins	Soluble in	Sources	Benefits	Notes
Vitamin D	Fat	Butterfat Eggs Organ meats Fish oils Adequate sunlight	Regulates absorption and utilization of calcium and phosphorus	Necessary for normal growth Deficiency link-to osteoporsis Synthetic sources can be toxic
Vitamin E	Fat	Nuts Seeds Unrefined vegetable oils Unrefined grains Legumes Leafy greens Butter	Circulation Tissue repair Healing Prevents polyunsaturated fatty acids from oxidizing	Works with trace minerals selenium and zinc to protect heart; high doses are not known to be toxic
Vitamin K	Fat	Dark leafy green vegetables	Normal blood clotting	Deficiency causes abnormal bleeding
Minerals	**Where found**	**Sources**	**Benefits**	**Notes**
Calcium	Most abundant mineral in the body Found in skeleton and teeth	Dairy products Leafy green vegetables Sea vegetables Sesame and sunflower seeds	Coagulates blood Monitors nerve impulses Maintains acid-alkaline balance in blood	Hormones, exercise, and diet affect how much is needed. Animal protein requires more calcium. Alcohol, sodas, and tobacco interfere with absorption.
Chloride	Primarily in hydrochloric acid in stomach	All plant foods Salt	Digestion Fluids inside and outside cells Acid-alkaline balance	Works with sodium and potassium
Magnesium	Tooth enamel	Dairy foods Sea vegetables Seafood Leafy greens	Enzyme reaction Carbohydrate and protein metabolism Acid-alkaline balance	Magnesium and calcium work together; their balance is important

Minerals	Soluble in	Sources	Benefits	Notes
Phosphorous	Second most abundant mineral in the body	Sea vegetables Whole grains Beans and legumes Nuts Seeds	Bones Kidney function Cells Acid-alkaline balance	Works with magnesium and calcium
Potassium and Sodium	Sodium in extra-cellular fluids Potassium in intra-cellular fluids	Potassium: vegetables and fruits Sodium: sea vegetables, salt, most processed foods	Cellular fluid balance Nerves Kidney function Muscle contraction and expansion Acid-alkaline balance	Potassium and sodium affect each other
Iron	Blood (red color)	Animal foods Prunes Figs Raisins Sea vegetables	Blood function Enzymatic activities	Inorganic iron can be toxic in excess
Iodine	Thyroid gland	Seafood Natural sea salt	Growth Metabolism	Too much or too little is hard on the body
Manganese	Bones	Whole grains Nuts Seeds Sea vegetables	Immune and nervous system	Involved in growth

◊ *Weight Loss and Gain*

Everyone carries some fat on their body. However, if you have more or less than what you want or what is ideal for your age and height, the excess or lack can cause health problems. Here are suggestions to help.

Losing Weight

1. Plan meals. Be proactive about what you will eat, rather than reactive or compulsive.
2. Eat breakfast. After fasting all night, eat something. Eat regularly through the day, so your body doesn't think it is starving and hang onto every calorie.
3. Satisfy sweet cravings with healthy carbohydrates more than desserts. Eat grains and chew them well. Eat sweet vegetables such as sweet potatoes and winter squash.
4. Sit for duration of meal, preferably at a table without a television on.
5. Drink water 15 minutes before the meal. Water adds moisture to the digestive tract and helps prevent overeating.
6. Take one bite of food and then put down the fork. Chew it and pay attention to how much you like it. When finished and not before, pick up fork and take the next bite. Many people position the fork over plate and gulp food, eager for the next bite without acknowledging the bite in the mouth.
7. Serve a beautiful, balanced, and adequate plate for yourself. Put enough food on the plate for a complete meal and avoid taking seconds. Present it like a restaurant does.
8. Have a healthy dessert. Eat fresh fruit, dried fruit and nuts, or homemade goods. Very few purchased baked goods are healthy, so make your own as much as possible.
9. When weather permits, take a 5 to 10 minute walk after eating. If you have eaten the right amount, your body will be grateful for the walk. If you have eaten too much, it is harder to walk. If you notice you are still hungry, either you haven't eaten enough or are experiencing cravings. If this is the case, drink water. Read the section on Cravings.
10. When weather prevents a walk, rise from the table and wash dishes. A little activity after eating stimulates digestion.
11. Enjoy your company. Feast on the interaction; eat one plate full, one bite at a time.
12. Pause before eating and say a blessing, either out loud or

silently. If you notice saliva in your mouth, smile. Your body is getting ready to eat.

Gaining Weight

1. Plan meals. Be proactive about calories and regular consumption. Choose smaller meals more often during the day in order to increase number of calories.
2. Eat breakfast. Don't skip any meals or fast. Eat healthy foods as often as possible.
3. Eat nutrient-dense foods, such as sweet potatoes, cooked vegetables, and chowders. Avoid dry and hard foods such as salads and crackers as they are harder to digest and encourage weight loss.
4. Eat soft and moist foods. Use beans in soups rather than refried, puddings rather than cookies, stewed fruits rather than dried, oats in porridge rather than granola. The moisture lubricates the digestive tract and provides a vehicle for heighted absorption.
5. Use supplements as needed. Probiotics before meals strengthen the digestive tract. Digestive enzymes after meals can enhance assimilation.

Appendix 5

◊ *Nutrition Menus*

These menus categorize individual items nutritionally into the macronutrients of complex carbohydrate (C), protein (P), and fats (F), and the micronutrients of vitamins and minerals (V+M). A food in parentheses indicates it is a secondary source of the nutrient; that food is the primary source of a different nutrient.

	Menu 1	**Menu 2**	**Menu 3**
C	Spanish rice (pinto beans) (corn chips)	Pita bread (hummus)	Brown rice
P	Pinto beans (cheese, if used)	Hummus, made with garbanzo beans	Tofu
F	Avocado Corn chips Cheese, if used (oil in fajita)	Tahini in hummus (oil in soup)	Oil in stir-fry
V+M	Fajita: onion, zucchini, pepper Salad Salsa (avocado) (tomato in rice)	Soup: cabbage, carrot, onion, celery, corn Salad toppings in pita: lettuce, sprouts	Vegetables: carrot, broccoli, water chestnuts, onion, ginger

◊ *Menus with Timings*

These menus estimate preparation time, if cooking for up to 4 people.

	10-minute menu 1 **Pancake Breakfast**	10-minute menu 2 **Rice Salad Lunch**	10-minute menu 3 **Pasta Dinner**
C	Pancakes	Brown rice, corn	Pasta with sauce
P	(egg in pancakes)	Chickpeas	(tofu in sauce)
F	Oil for frying	Olive oil in dressing	Olive oil in sauce
V+M	Berries	Carrot, celery, onion, cucumber, umeboshi vinegar	Vegetable stir-fry with tofu and juices thickened for sauce
Notes	Add miso soup for 15 minute prep	Use cooked rice, corn, and chickpeas to save time	Tomato sauce is also quick

	30-minute menu 1 **Crepes for Brunch**	30-minute menu 2 **Pasta Dinner**	30-minute menu 3 **Rice and Bean Dinner**
C	Crepes	Pasta	White rice
P	(tofu in veg filling) (egg in crepe)	Tempeh	Pinto beans
F	Oil for frying crepes and sautéing filling	Oil for frying Pesto	Oil for sautéing vegetables
V+M	Broccoli, garlic, carrot, onion, etc.	Greens Sweet potatoes	Stir-fry carrot, peas, onion, etc.
Notes	Cut vegetables in small pieces for best results; cutting takes more time	More dishes take more time than 10-minute pasta dinner	Beans in slow cooker all day shorten prep time; white rice is quick

	60-minute menu 1 **Quinoa Salad Lunch**	60-minute menu 2 **Fish Dinner**	60-minute menu 3 **Soup and Quick Bread Dinner**
C	Quinoa	Couscous Cookie	Cornbread or corn muffins
P	Red lentils	Salmon	Black bean soup
F	(olive oil in dressing)	(oil in salad dressing) (oil in cookie) (fat in fish)	(oil in cornbread)
V+M	Peas, carrot, celery, red onion, umeboshi vinegar	Broccoli Salad	Salad (vegetables in soup)
Notes	Red lentils are fastest cooking bean	Couscous and vegetables can be combined as a pilaf; omit dessert and shorten prep time	Use cooked beans to make soup

Time	1½-hour menu **Meal with brown rice**	2-hour menu **Meal with baked vegetables**	3-hour menu **Meal with boiled beans**
C	Brown rice	Brown rice	Brown rice
P	Red lentils	Azuki beans or brown lentils	Pinto or black beans
F	Nuts	Seeds	Seeds
V+M	Any vegetables sautéed or simmered	Baked squash	Any vegetables
Notes	Brown rice requires about 1 hour of cooking no matter what else is prepared	Azuki beans and lentils take about 1½ hours of cooking; baked vegetables take about 1 hour	Pinto and black beans take about 2 hours to boil

◊ *Celebration Menus*

These menus offer examples of menus for special occasions. Timing for these menus often is different from everyday cooking, as special dishes require extra time.

	Menu 1 **Birthday Meal**	Menu 2 **Vegetarian Holiday**	Menu 3 **Animal Food Holiday**
C	Croquettes (cooked millet and flour)	Brown rice pilaf Sweet potatoes Rolls	White rice Mashed potatoes Rolls
P	(chickpeas in croquette)	Seitan or tofu main dish	Turkey
F	Oil for frying Sauce for croquette	Tahini sauce Spread for rolls Olive oil in dressing	Gravy Spread for rolls Olive oil in dressing
V+M	Salad	Broccoli Salad	Broccoli Salad
Dessert	Birthday cake	Apple pie	Pumpkin pie Cranberry relish
Notes	Items can be prepared in advance	Brown rice complements vegetarian protein	White rice complements animal protein

◊ *Cultural Menus*

These menus highlight the grains and beans that various cultures have traditionally eaten in combination. While actual menus are more elaborate than what is listed, you can use this list as a model from which to begin. Cultural menus are traditional sources of nutrition, local foods, and complementary tastes. Refer to any ethnic cookbook for more ideas.

Culture	Grain (C) and bean (P)	Rest of meal (F and V+M)
Mexico	Corn and pinto beans Rice and pinto beans	Vegetables such as peppers, tomatoes, zucchini, cucumbers, garlic, etc.
Japan	Rice and azuki beans Rice and soybean products	Miso soup Tempura vegetables such as sweet potato and broccoli Norimaki sushi Burdock in vegetable dishes
India	Rice and dhal (lentils) Rice and garbanzo beans	Vegetables such as cauliflower and potato Spices such as cumin and turmeric and mustard Cucumber in dishes
Middle East	Pita and garbanzo beans Couscous and garbanzo beans	Sesame seed tahini Vegetables such as lettuce, tomato, and cucumber
Northern Europe	Rye bread and pea soup Wheat bread and beans Oats and seeds	Vegetables such as cabbage and turnip
Italy	Pasta and fava beans Pasta and white beans	Vegetables such as cucumber, tomato, etc.

◊ *Intuition about Sprouts*

Source. Sprouts provide a vitality of new growth and nutrition different than their source.

Shopping. Buy organic sprouts as fresh as possible and use within a day or so. However, once you learn to sprout your own, you may never buy again, as it is quite easy and inexpensive. Buy organic seeds for sprouting.

Measuring. Use about 1 tablespoon of seeds in a 4-cup jar for sprouting. Other containers can be used too with similar proportions.

Timing. Sprouts are done on various schedules. A warm room speeds the process. Sprouts are ready to eat when the first two leaves appear.

Intuitive tip. Growing sprouts is an easy way to experience intuition. Start with what you will use. Get equipment together. Rinse daily and more often if very hot. Rinse water is good for houseplants.

Recipes

1. *Clover or alfalfa sprouts*. Soak about a tablespoon of seeds in ample water overnight in a 4 cup jar. Secure cheesecloth on top of jar with rubber bands. Drain by tipping jar upside down. Rinse daily; don't let cheesecloth become totally dry. Watch the sprouts for 3 to 5 days and eat when the first two leaves appear.

2. *Mung or lentil sprouts*. Watch for the hull of seed to detach.

3. *Rice*. Soak rice for 1 to 2 days, watch for first signs of sprouting, and then cook.

◊ *Intuition about Fermented Foods*

Source. Miso, soy sauce, umeboshi, vinegar, pickles.

Shopping. These fermented foods are usually bought ready-to-eat. Traditionally, ingredients were held for a period of time and changed into a beneficial health-giving, enzyme-rich product. Currently, these traditional products are still available. Unfortunately, many companies have developed short cuts to provide these items in less time. For example, traditional soy sauce requires 2 to 3 years; a quick soy sauce is ready in 2 to 3 months. When you buy any of these items, look for labels from reputable companies and ingredients without alcohol. Some labels state how long the item was aged. All of these items can be taste-tested for quality.

Miso. Miso is made from soybeans and a grain, such as barley or brown rice. Some kinds have only soybeans or are made from white rice, azuki beans, or chickpeas. Miso is fermented 1 to 3 years, depending on kind. It is usually used to season soup and is added right before eating, without boiling. Taste a small amount on tongue or dilute in small amount of water. Traditional miso tastes delicious and pleasing.

Soy sauce. Soy sauce is made from soybeans and wheat; some varieties are wheat-free. Soy sauce is used in cooking to season foods, usually right before eating. It has less sodium than salt. Taste a few drops on the tongue, or dilute in small amount of water. Traditional soy sauce tastes delicious and satisfying. Inferior soy sauce tastes harsh.

Umeboshi. Umeboshi is a salted preserved plum, a special variety of plum originating in Japan. Traditional umeboshi is fermented 2 to 3 years. The taste is salty, sour, and somewhat sweet. Umeboshi is often eaten with rice or used in teas, as it is reported to help digestion. The brine, called umeboshi vinegar, is not a true vinegar, but a salty, sour liquid that is delicious in dressings and sauces. To taste umeboshi, sample a small amount or dilute in water.

Vinegar. Traditional vinegars are aged like wine, in big barrels that allow flavors to deepen and develop. Many kinds are available— apple cider, brown rice, and balsamic are a few. All can be used in dressings or at the end of cooking. Look for quality products from reputable sources and with an ingredient list free of alcohol. To taste, sample a small amount for flavor. Superior vinegars have appeal. Inferior vinegars taste harsh.

Pickles. Naturally made pickles aid digestion. Look for sauerkraut, kimchi, or pickles made without alcohol, sugars, preservatives, or pasteurization.

Measuring. Use naturally fermented foods and/or products often, every day if your health allows. See recipes below for suggested amounts.

Timing 1. Timing is important in the original preparation for success in fermentation. If you make pickles, allow enough time and monitor the timing.

Timing 2. Timing is important in using fermented foods in cooking. Fermented foods are best used without boiling so as to preserve the active enzymes. Cooking destroys enzymes.

Intuitive tips. Taste products, as per suggestions above.

Recipes

    1. *Miso soup*. Miso can be added to any soup. Ladle hot soup

into bowl and add about 1 teaspoon of miso per serving. Stir to dilute. Soups with other seasonings need less miso. Alternately, to make miso soup, boil water, add cut vegetables and boil until soft, then turn heat off and add miso. There are many ingredients that make delicious miso soup; try carrots, cabbage, tofu, fresh corn, and daikon radish. Garnish with cut scallions.

2. *Umeboshi kuzu drink.* Bring 1 cup of water, 1 umeboshi plum, and 1 teaspoon of kuzu powder to boil. Simmer for a few minutes, then add up to 1 teaspoon of soy sauce. This drink is reputed to help digestion and strengthen the digestive tract. Kuzu is a starch from the kuzu plant and is said to help the intestines.

3. *Chinese cabbage pickles.* Cut about 4 cups of cabbage leaves into shreds. Mix well with 1 to 2 tablespoons of sea salt. For spicy pickles, add 1 tablespoon each of crushed garlic, finely minced fresh ginger root, and chili pepper. Pack into clean quart jar and press down to help cabbage release its juices. Ferment 3 days or until cabbage changes in flavor.

4. *All-purpose dressing.* Mix 4 parts olive oil, 1 part balsamic vinegar, 1 part soy sauce, and 1 part brown rice vinegar for a delicious dressing good on pastas and vegetables. Add herbs and spices of choice.

Appendix 6

◊ *Intuition about Sweeteners and Desserts*

Source. Desserts provide an end to a meal and satisfy emotional needs.

Shopping. Buy quality fruits, sweeteners, oils, and flours to prepare desserts. If you purchase ready-to-eat desserts, buy the best available. Unfortunately, most desserts contain inferior oils, and many contain sugar or its derivatives. If, like me, you give up after reading labels, buy nuts and fresh or dried fruit to serve the easiest and simplest dessert possible.

Sweeteners. There are a vast number of sweeteners, ranging from artificial and highly processed ones to natural sweeteners that are minimally processed. While everyone loves the sweet taste, too much is detrimental. And, artificial sweeteners can have a disastrous effect on the body, especially if over-consumed.

Let your intuition help you learn how to satisfy your desire for sweetness without harm. While many lessons in this book are devoted to this theme, here are specific ideas for using sweeteners. Avoid artificial ones. Buy natural ones, but be selective because some are better than others. Natural sugars are marketed under many names and labels: honey, agave, maple syrup, brown rice syrup, stevia, and other natural sweeteners.

A simple taste test can alert you to sweeteners that are over stimulating and ones that are comfortable, both in flavor and how you react. Just sample a small amount and notice your response.

Sugar is a broad term for glucose, a simple molecule that enters the bloodstream and feeds the brain. Some sources provide glucose instantly and produce a "sugar high," characterized by increased alertness and energy, followed by a "sugar low" of less energy. The healthiest sweeteners are ones that provide glucose in a gentler manner. Brown rice syrup and maple syrup are my sweeteners of choice with honey as a third option, especially for guests who have a sweet tooth. To heighten your taste awareness overall, avoid all sugar for 10 days; your tongue will become more sensitive to all other flavors.

Sugar is an addictive substance and can mask intuition. I urge you to devote time to developing intuition by avoiding sugar for at least some period of time.

Measuring. Some desserts don't require measuring. Others are contingent on proportions. For these items, use recipes unless and until you are comfortable making desserts without measuring.

Timing. Baked desserts need thorough cooking. Use recipes to help you gauge when items are done. This helps you be familiar with the final product so you can adjust accordingly when you have a different stove, pans, elevation, or temperatures. Then you can do something out of the ordinary, such as bake a dessert in a cast-iron Dutch oven over coals at high altitude, after noticing you forgot a watch!

Intuitive Tips
1. Notice proportion of dry ingredients to liquid ingredients.
2. Notice proportion of sweeteners and fat to other liquid and dry ingredients.
3. Notice proportion of salt and leavening to flour and other dry ingredients.
4. Generally, dry ingredients are mixed or sifted together, and liquid ingredients are mixed together separately. Then dry

and wet are mixed together.

5. Procedures are standard too. Preheat oven, often to 350 degrees. Prepare bakeware. Mix dry. Mix wet. Mix together. Bake until lightly browned and done in center.

6. Consistency of batter before baking should be consistent with standard recipes—not too wet or dry. Baking is not rocket science. If you have baked before, you will feel comfortable.

7. A little salt makes desserts taste better.

8. Liquid sweeteners need to be included with the liquids.

9. Use quality fats in baking. Liquid oils break down at temperatures in excess of 212 degrees F. Use organic unrefined extra virgin coconut oil for baking.

Recipes

1. *Dried fruit and nuts, no cooking.* Try dates and almonds.

2. *Stewed fruits and compotes.* No measuring. Simmer dried apricots in water with dried ginger, coriander, or lemon zest until soft. Experiment with other fruits and flavorings.

3. *Fruit sauces.* No measuring. Cut fresh apples and cook into applesauce. Add salt and cinnamon. Experiment with other fresh fruits or combinations.

4. *Try making a dessert you have made before without measuring.* Assemble the same ingredients and eyeball the amounts. This can be fun and satisfying. Many desserts are easy to improvise, such as cobblers or pie fillings, and many cooks adapt readily. Take the next step and intuit more of the recipe.

◊ *Food Combining Menus*

All menus combine foods—some for taste, some for health. Some combinations are based on how digestion works; others depend on individual responses to various foods. The following two groups of menus represent two general food-combining categories: 1) Simple and 2) Full with fermented foods included.

The first group follows simple food-combining ideas:

1. Carbohydrates (C) and proteins (P) are served at separate meals.

2. Fruits (vitamins and minerals; V+M) are served alone.

3. There are a minimal number of foods served at one time.

4. Vegetables (V+M) are encouraged. Fats (F) are in small amounts.

These menus are practical for anyone with delicate digestion or during times of fasting, coming off a fast, or recovering from illness. If a person desires to lose weight, these menus can give a framework for other menus. The key is: B=Breakfast, L=Lunch, S=Snack, D=Dinner.

Light Menus				
	Few calories, little protein, low fat	Nutrition spaced through day	Appropriate during high fever	Appropriate during recovery or when person is cold and weak
B	Oatmeal (C)	Blueberries and strawberries (V+M)	Vegetable soup (V+M)	Miso soup (V+M)
L	Salad with seeds	Rice (C) and veg-etables (V+M)	Soft rice (rice porridge) (C)	Soft rice (C) Cooked vege-tables (V+M)
S	Fruit (F, V+M)	Nuts (F)	Steamed vege-tables (V+M)	Soft rice (C)
D	Steamed vege-tables (V+M)	Lentil soup (P) Salad with lemon (V+M)	Vegetable soup with noodles (C, V+M)	Chicken soup (P, F, V+M)

The second group highlights fermented foods. Food combining ideas include:

1. Complex carbohydrates (C) and plant-based protein (P) are served at each meal.

2. Fermented food (FR) is served.

3. Vegetables (V+M) and fats (F) are included.

These menus are samples of full meals that contain fermented foods and are useful any time. This list outlines specific meals.

Full Breakfast	Full Lunch	Full Dinner 1	Full Dinner 2
Miso soup with tofu (P, V+M) Brown rice (C) Daikon pickle (FR)	Norimake sushi of: Nori (V+M) Brown rice (C) Umeboshi (FR) Avocado (F) Carrot (V+M) Ginger pickle (FR) Fried tempeh (P, F)	Miso soup (V+M) Sandwich of: Naturally-leavened bread (C) Fried tempeh (P, F) Mustard (Flavor) Sauerkraut (FR)	Brown rice (C) Dhal (curried lentils) (P) Stir-fried vege-tables (V+M, F) Yogurt (FR)

◊ *Discharges*

The healing process can initiate temporary symptoms that may be uncomfortable. Discharges (detoxing) can happen as the body adjusts and purges itself of unwanted physical matter and toxins. Usually the body seeks to rid these through the easiest channels—the digestive tract, lungs, and skin.

During my first and second years of changing my diet, I experienced discharges. On occasion, I had stomachaches, coughs, putrid eliminations, skin rashes, and nasal secretions. I also stopped menstruating for a period of time. Each of these symptoms cleared after a brief bout.

Not everyone experiences such adjustments. However, if you do, there are some good things to know so that you don't worry. First, a discharge is a clearing process. Even though it can be uncomfortable, it is the body's way of getting better. Unless the symptoms are unbearable, let them run their course.

The second thing to know is that symptoms of discharge can be similar to symptoms of illness. The difference is that in sickness, the body is often dealing with diseases or germs. There are a few ways to tell if the symptom is from a discharge rather than a sickness. The ideas here are general:

1. *Appetite, no appetite, nausea.* When a person is sick, often there is no appetite. With discharge, often there is an appetite. Sometimes, there is a deep, sick-to-the-stomach feeling. If you are experiencing symptoms, consider your appetite. For example, when I had skin rashes and cracked fingers, I had an appetite, although certain foods (notably tomatoes) aggravated the discomfort. When I had stomachaches, I had no appetite until later in the day after all the food had passed through my system. When I am sick, I have no appetite until the illness is gone.

2. *Sleep, no sleep, restlessness.* When a person is sick, often there is restlessness and/or fitful sleep. If you are experiencing symptoms, consider how you sleep. With discharge, a person can usually sleep. For example, when I had coughs, skin problems, and lost my period, I slept well. However, when one cough turned into bronchitis, my sleep was affected.

3. *Energy, vitality, exhaustion.* When a person is sick, often there is lack of energy. With discharge, energy may or may not be different. If you are experiencing symptoms, consider your level of vitality. During some of my stomachaches, I felt exhausted. But after they passed as putrid eliminations, I regained my energy.

4. *Time, duration of symptoms.* When a person is sick, often he or she has an internal guide for how long it should last. If you are experiencing symptoms, consider the length of time they have lasted and your level of discomfort. Some symptoms can be allowed to run their course while others need intervention. For example, I let a 1- or 2-day runny nose run its course. However, one time the symptoms lasted 4 days and progressed into bronchitis; I consulted someone.

I also went to a gynecologist after my period had ceased for a couple of months.

5. *Gut feeling, okay or not okay.* When you have symptoms, often you have a gut or an intuitive feeling that something out of the ordinary is going on. What do you do? Some people run to the doctor for everything. Some people refuse to go to the doctor for anything. Decide which course you usually take and then reassess whether this time the symptoms merit a different course of action. This is relying on your intuition and listening to your gut.

Overall, establish some parameters about your intuition when your body signals it needs attention. Listen to your body. Apply common sense to what you are comfortable dealing with, and consult others as needed. While discharges are the way the body heals, do not assume all discomfort is a discharge. At the same time, do not assume every level of discomfort requires medical attention.

Please don't try to diagnose yourself if you have any doubts at all. It is better to consult someone and find out you're okay rather than suffer and have something serious develop.

Intuition is not a substitute for medical advice. Intuition is an inner knowing that urges you to take care of yourself, and this includes seeking medical care when required.

Practice inner awareness each time you experience discomfort; you will strengthen your intuitive ability to help yourself.

Appendix 7

◊ *Intuition about Leftovers*

Source. People often have sharply divided feeling about leftovers—either hate them or love them. While certain foods and dishes make good leftovers and are practical and timesaving, others don't. Specifically, dishes such as lasagna, soup, and muffins are great the next day. Single items such as cooked brown rice or garbanzo beans are easy to use again by incorporating into new dishes. Other foods, notably green vegetables, take a turn for the worse as leftovers. Keep them fresh for best appeal. Here are other tips.

Intuitive tips

1. Reheating. To reheat leftovers and retain original texture and flavor, use a complementary process. Heat casseroles and muffins in the oven, dip pasta in hot water, and simmer soup on the stovetop. A simple way to reheat single servings of food is to place over steam. Either place servings in a steamer basket, or place items on a heat-resistant plate and set plate on a large bamboo steamer tray. There is considerable debate on the effects of microwaves on health. I avoid them because I believe the radiation from a microwave oven changes the molecular structure of foods. If you do use a microwave, I recommend limiting the frequency and duration of use.

2. Transition foods. Include leftover ingredients into a new

dish. Cooked grains, pasta, and beans make wonderful one-pot meals.

3. Quantity and advance planning. Prepare grains and beans in quantities for more than one meal in order to have intentional leftovers. This step is helpful for certain dishes that require multiple steps. Of all the vegetables, winter squash is most amenable to advance preparation.

Recipes

1. *Fried rice.* Sauté vegetables and seasonings until done. Add already cooked brown rice to heat through. Try garlic, ginger, curry, onion, carrot, peas, tofu, soy sauce.

2. *Pasta skillet.* Sauté vegetables and seasonings until done. Add already cooked pasta and beans to heat through. Add sauce. Try garlic, onions, peppers, broccoli or cabbage, corn, cooked garbanzo beans, and a sauce of tomato and basil or tahini and basil.

3. *Fried polenta.* Make polenta one day and scoop into loaf pan to set. When cool (or next day) turn out of pan, slice into servings, fry, and serve.

◊ *Intuition about Eating Out*

Everyone goes out to eat occasionally. Even those who cook all their own food long for restaurants with the same quality they have at home. Here are some tips for navigating restaurants.

1. *Social needs.* Many times people eat out with friends, and if this is the case, enjoy the camaraderie first, food second.

2. *Quality assurance.* Restaurants have a standard of quality that may be different from what you have at home. The quality may be in ethnic flavors, certain chef, location, or in the deal-of-the-day. You can identify this quality by what is advertised. Perhaps the restaurant features organic produce, fresh-caught fish, or authentic cuisine. Take advantage of the best the restaurant offers. The flip side of this idea is that quality can be less than ideal too. Unless you are certain of the integrity of the kitchen, assume that items are not organic. The quality of oils, salt, and dairy foods are especially important.

3. *Things you don't want.* Note things you don't want to eat at all. For me, this is meat, MSG, and white refined sugar. Also realize that most restaurants use more fat and salt in food than you do at home. Select foods with lower amounts of fat. For example, avoid deep-fried items. Look for low quantities of dairy and butter. Request that salad dressings be served on the side. Realize that dairy is hidden in many soups and desserts, and anything that contains mayonnaise has extra fat. Animal foods and stocks show up in refried beans and soups, so ask if you have any questions.

4. *Things you want.* Look for what you consider healthy, such as selections with enough vegetables or where grains are incorporated. Many restaurants offer vegetarian selections; Thai and Indian restaurants often serve beans and tofu, good sources of protein. Italian and Japanese restaurants often have fish. Navigate the meat selections and aim for adequate vegetables.

5. *Small portions.* Remember to chew well at restaurants and savor the flavors and experiences. If portions are large, which they usually are, share with your friends or take home the extra. One technique is to mentally divide your plate in half and eat only that portion.

Resources

Aihara, Herman. *Basic Macrobiotics*. George Ohsawa Macrobiotic Foundation, 1998. *www.OhsawaMacrobiotics.com*.

Batmanghelidg, F., M.D. *Your Body's Many Cries for Water*. Global Health Solutions. Inc., 2008. *www.watercure.com*.

Barnard, Neal, M.D. *Dr. Neal Barnard's Program for Reversing Diabetes*. Rodale Books, 2008. *www.nealbarnard.org* or *www.pcrm.org*.

Brown, Simon. *Macrobiotics for Life*. North Atlantis Books, 2009. *Modern-Day Macrobiotics*. North Atlantis Books, 2007. *www.chienergy.co.uk*.

Campbell, T. Colin. *The China Study*. BonBella Books, 2006. *www.thechinastudy.com*.

Colbin, Annemarie. *Food and Healing*. Ballantine, 1986. *The Whole-Foods Guide to Strong Bones*. New Harbinger Publications, 2009. *www.foodandhealing.com*.

Cousens, Gabriel, M.D. *Spiritual Nutrition*. North Atlantis Books, 2005. *www.treeoflife.nu*.

D'Adamo, Peter J. *Eat Right For Your Type*. Putnam Adult, 1997. *www.dadamo.com*.

Enig, Mary G. *Know Your Fats*. Bethesda Press, 2000. *www.westonprice.org*.

Esselstyn, Caldwell B., Jr. *Prevent and Reverse Heart Disease*. Avery Trade, 2008. *www.heartattackproof.com.*

Fallon, Sally. *Nourishing Traditions*. New Trends Publishing, 2001. *www.westonprice.org.*

Ferré, Carl. *Essential Guide to Macrobiotics*. George Ohsawa Macrobiotic Foundation, 2011. *www.OhsawaMacrobiotics.com.*

Kotzsch,Ronald E., Ph.D. *Macrobiotics Beyond Food*. Japan Publications. 1988.

Kushi, Michio and Alex Jack. *The Macrobiotic Path to Total Health*. Ballantine Books, 2004. *www.michiokushi.org.*

Lechasseur, Eric and Sanae Suzuki. *Love, Eric and Sanae*. Mugan, LLC., 2007. *www.loveericinc.com.*

McCarty, Meredith. *Sweet and Natural*. St. Martin's Press, 2001. *www.healingcuisine.com.*

McDougall, John, M.D. and Mary McDougall. *The Starch Solution*. Rodale Books, 2012. *The McDougall Program*. Plume, 1991. *www.drmcdougall.com.*

Morgan, Christy. *Blissful Bites*. BenBella Books, 2011. *www.blissfulchef.com.*

Ohsawa, George with Carl Ferré. *Essential Ohsawa*. George Ohsawa Macrobiotic Foundation, 2002. *www.OhsawaMacrobiotics.com.*

Ong, Julie. *The Everything Guide to Macrobiotics*. Adams Media, 2010. *www.juliesong.com.*

Pirello, Christina. *Cooking the Whole Foods Way*. HP Trade, 2007. *www.christinacooks.com.*

Porter, Jessica. *The Hip Chick's Guide to Macrobiotics*. Avery, 2004. *www.hipchicksmacrobiotics.com.*

Robbins, John and Dean Ornish, M.D. *The Food Revolution*. Conari Press, 2010. *www.ornishspectrum.com*.

Robbins, John. *Diet for a New America*. HJ Kramer, 1998. www.*johnrobbins.info*.

Shelton, Herbert M. *Food Combining Made Easy*. Book Pubishing Company, 2012. *www.soilandhealth.org*.

Stanchich, Lino. *Power Eating Program*. Health Products, Inc., 19989. *www.greatlifeglobal.com*.

Stec, Laura and Eugene Cordero, PhD. *Cool Cuisine*. Gibbs Smith, 2008. *www.laurastec.com*.

Turner, Kristina. *The Self-Healing Cookbook*. Earthtones Press, 2002.

Varona, Verne. *Macrobiotics for Dummies*. For Dummies, 2009. *www.vernevarona.com*.

Waxman, Melanie. *Eat Me Now!* PublishAmerica, 2008. *www.celebrate4health.com*.

Weil, Andrew, M.D. *Eating Well for Optimum Health*. William Morrow Paperbacks, 2001. *www.drweil.com*.

Wood, Rebecca. *The New Whole Foods Encyclopedia*. Penguin, 2010. *www.rebeccawood.com*.

About the Author

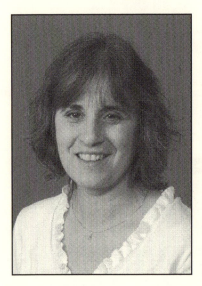

JULIA FERRÉ is a certified hypnotherapist, specializing in past life regression, and a Reiki master. She lectures and counsels, offering sessions for energy, attunement, and personal growth, throughout the world. In addition to the *Food and Intuition 101* series, she is author of *Basic Macrobiotic Cooking* and *French Meadows Cookbook*.

Julia lives in California with husband Carl and their four sons. For more information, see: *www. JuliaFerre.com.*

Other Books from the
George Ohsawa Macrobiotic Foundation

Acid Alkaline Companion - Carl Ferré; 2009; 121 pp.
Acid and Alkaline - Herman Aihara; 1986; 121 pp.
As Easy As 1, 2, 3 - Pamela Henkel and Lee Koch; 1990; 176 pp.
Basic Macrobiotic Cooking, 20th Anniversary Edition - Julia
    Ferré; 2007; 275 pp.
Book of Judo - George Ohsawa; 1990; 150 pp.
Cancer and the Philosophy of the Far East - George Ohsawa;
    1981; 165 pp.
Cooking with Rachel - Rachel Albert; 1989; 328 pp.
Essential Guide to Macrobiotics - Carl Ferré; 2011; 131 pp.
Essential Ohsawa - George Ohsawa, edited by Carl Ferré; 1994;
    238 pp.
French Meadows Cookbook - Julia Ferré; 2008; 275 pp.
Macrobiotics: An Invitation to Health and Happiness - George
    Ohsawa; 1971; 128 pp.
Naturally Healthy Gourmet - Margaret Lawson with Tom Monte;
    1994; 232 pp.
Philosophy of Oriental Medicine - George Ohsawa; 1991; 153 pp.
Practical Guide to Far Eastern Macrobiotic Medicine - George
    Ohsawa; 2010; 279 pp.
Zen Cookery - G.O.M.F.; 1985; 140 pp.
Zen Macrobiotics, Unabridged Edition - George Ohsawa, edited
    by Carl Ferré; 1995; 206 pp.

A wide selection of macrobiotic books is available from the George
Ohsawa Macrobiotic Foundation, P.O. Box 3998, Chico, CA 95965;
530-566-9765. Order toll free: 800-232-2372. Or, you may visit
www.OhsawaMacrobiotics.com for all books and PDF downloads
of many books.